The Milk Soy Protein Intolerance (MSPI) Guidebook/Cookbook

Tamara Field

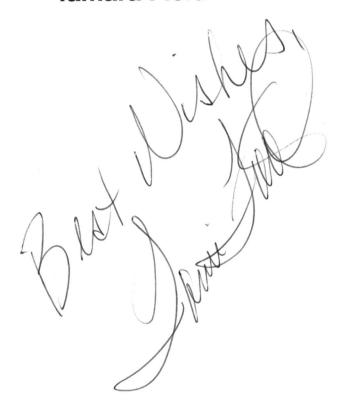

VANTAGE PRESS
New York

The recipes contained herein have not been tested by the publisher.

FIRST EDITION

Copyright © 2001 by Tamara Field

Published by Vantage Press, Inc.
516 West 34th Street, New York, New York 10001

Manufactured in the United States of America
ISBN: 0-533-13841-8

Library of Congress Catalog Card No.: 00-91263

0 9 8 7 6 5 4 3 2 1

To "my boys":

My husband, Larry for this idea and the love and encouragement it took to make this book happen and to keep me motivated when I lost confidence in my own ideas. I thank you also for sharing rice milk with me and eating everything I made and make, and being honest about how much you like or dislike my creations. Yes, you are right; most of the dishes would have been "better if you could only add a little cheese."

To Max, my now three-and-a-half-year-old, thanks for *usually* eating what I made for dinner, and understanding (or maybe not understanding) when I needed to hold and feed your little brother when I knew you wanted my arms and attention for yourself. Please know that it was our struggles with your digestive system that introduced me to the wonderful world of MSPI. You are such a happy, bright, and sensitive little boy . . . I'll love you forever.

To Natie, who experienced this diet firsthand, via me. What a pleasure it was to be able to nurse you for a year. I am so fortunate that this diet gave me the opportunity to experience motherhood to its fullest in loving you that way. You are the most sweet, cuddly, and carefree and independent little boy; you know exactly what you want, and that you want it now! My love for you is also forever and always.

Contents

Foreword

Milk Soy Protein Intolerance is commonly acknowledged and diagnosed by both pediatricians and family physicians. In the medical field this occurrence is also known as eosinophilic gastroenteritis. MSPI is diagnosed through the history of an infant with irritability (colic-like behavior), poor growth, abnormal stools; some of which visibly show blood. Confirmation of the diagnosis is often made by a biopsy of the intestinal tissue showing an increased amount of eosinophilic cells, eroded intestinal villi, and hemorrhagic tissue. An increase in the level of eosinophilic cells may also correlate with an allergic response of the intestinal tissues due to the introduction of an allergic compound. Many physicians request that parents alter the infant's formula or the mother's diet (for breastfed infants) prior to having a gastroenterologist perform an invasive biopsy, then if the symptoms diminish, or even cease, the diagnosis of MSPI is assumed.

Both formula-fed and breast-fed infants can develop an intolerance to cow's milk protein and also soy protein. For infants fed with formula, it is easy to change to a different formula, but more specialized formulas are more expensive. For many families the costs of these formulas are prohibitive. For an infant who is breastfed, the mother's diet must be altered to avoid milk and soy proteins in order to continue breastfeeding. This approach is certainly a less costly solution to the dietary demands of an MSPI infant.

As a pediatrician who suspects MSPI, I first advise the breastfeeding mother to eliminate all dairy products from her diet; then if the infant's symptoms decrease, I advise the mother to continue with the dietary restrictions. If these measures help, but the infant is still fussy, irritable, or having blood-streaked stools, then I also suggest removing soy products from the mother's diet. To date, I have had only one handout to give to mothers on the dietary restrictions for MSPI. This consisted of a list of the following foods: plain fruit, vegetables, meats, a certain type of French bread, and a list of ingredients to be avoided on the MSPI diet. All packaged or processed items with milk or soy proteins must be eliminated. I cannot imagine what hope I offered to these mothers as I sent them out of my office.

This book offers a realistic approach to MSPI and the breastfeeding mother's dietary restrictions. This guidebook and cookbook goes beyond offering the standard information about MSPI; it offers guidance on products, manufacturers, and foods or products that may be substituted for those commonly used items that must be avoided on this diet. In addition, it offers support and knowledge to the mother who must make the immediate and drastic changes necessary in her diet to continue breastfeeding her infant and easing the symptoms of MSPI.

Monique L. Macklem, M.D.

Author's Note

Dr. Macklem is a fellow of the American Academy of Pediatricians and also an Associate Professor of Pediatrics at Creighton University in Omaha.

Acknowledgments

I have many people to thank for their inspiration and kindness in helping me with this project. First, I must thank my mother. I grew up in a house filled with wonderful smells, and they always came from my mother's kitchen. Fresh baked bread, homemade soups, cookies, casseroles and produce fresh from her garden (which she made me weed, by the way) are all part of my very fondest childhood memories. Also, Mom, thanks for trying many of these recipes out for me and giving me your insights. You've always supported me wholeheartedly in anything I ever pursued. So, Mom, thanks for teaching me how to bake and cook, and for making me the 'foodaholic' that I am today.

And, in thanking my mother, I also must thank my grandmother, from whom many of my mother's talents come. I remember the smells of freshly-baked fruitbread, passed on from her mother, Helga, and the many candies and cookies that were plentiful during the winter holidays and most other times of the year (if you knew where to look!). Grandma, you still make the best date pinwheel cookies I have ever eaten! I didn't include them in this cookbook because I can't make them nearly as good as you!

Many thanks to our pediatrician, Monique Macklem, who was so incredibly attentive when Max was born, helping us sort out all of his digestive problems. She refused to call his incessant crying 'colic' until we had investigated every other possibility. At seven weeks we went, at her referral, to a gastroenterologist who diagnosed Max with MSPI. I am so grateful for your care and concern over the past three-and-a-half years, I cannot imagine having a more supportive, knowledgeable, and caring physician to care for our children. Thank you so much.

With our thanks to Dr. Macklem, go my thanks to her partner, Steve Sindelar M.D. I remember a few teary moments (or hours) that he talked me through when Dr. Macklem had time off. You've always been very caring and taken excellent care of our boys, as well.

To my friend, Linda, many thanks for all your support and love. You would always try recipes and report back to me rave reviews and any mistakes I made. I thank you for being so honest and such a true friend.

To Sharon Novak, our day-care provider, thank you for loving my children, and caring for them when I needed time to work on this book, and my many other jobs! Thank you for always being so encouraging and never judgmental about the extra time I took to get things done. I can't imagine ever having a better place for our children to be.

To Kathryn Heldt, a registered dietitian at Children's Hospital in Omaha, who gave me advice on details of this diet that no one else could have given. Thank you for being so kind and available for my questions.

Thanks also to Gretchen Thomas, a dear friend, advice-giver, and superb mother. Thank you for trying recipes for me, for loving our family so much, and being a constant source of encouragement and good wishes.

Another source of affirmation and encouragement was my hairdresser, Merrilyn. Thanks for the great haircuts (and highlights!) and hours of sharing life, emotions, and ideas that made me feel like I could do anything. I am surrounded by so many people who are so positive and encouraging and I highly recommend it! I can draw strength from so many sources when needed. Thank you, Merrilyn, for being one of those people!

I must say thank you to a few others as well, who continually inquired and encouraged me in my efforts with this book. To Mark and Jill, who have been there through all our life events and have been such wonderful friends—thank you! To Beth, mommy to Alexandra, who is betrothed to one of my sons, you are a dear friend and beautiful singer; thanks for the friendship and encouragement. To Jayne, thanks for trying my recipes, and Todd, thanks for eating them!

Finally to so many other friends and colleagues, whether in my nursing or music world. If I name you all, I will forget someone. All the seemingly small comments of encouragement, or just the fact that you would ask "How's the cookbook coming?" meant a great deal! Thank you all.

Introduction

I first heard of Milk Soy Protein Intolerance (MSPI) in January of 1997 at the office of a pediatric gastroenterologist who had just performed a proctosigmoidoscopy and biopsy on my seven-week-old son. He told me that Max's digestive problem was MSPI and that it would be much easier for me if I stopped breastfeeding now and put him on a special formula. Of course, at that moment my head was spinning. I had finally found out the reason my son had been screaming the first seven weeks of his life and though I wanted to continue breastfeeding, I did not want to cause him anymore pain. The doctor told me that there was a diet I could follow to continue breastfeeding, but that it was very difficult to follow. Wanting to make the best choice for my son, I stopped breastfeeding that day and started him on formula.

In retrospect, the doctor was right, even though I regret that I did not continue breastfeeding; with the demands of a new infant, and trying to figure out a complicated diet, I might have gone mad. I knew though, that if I had any more children, I would try any diet possible in order to breastfeed. So, during the first few months of my pregnancy with my second son, Nate, I began preparing for the MSPI diet.

Determined that I would not lack for good things to eat, and that I *would* find chocolate that was acceptable on this diet, I started shopping. Little by little, I found many acceptable alternatives for much of the food I enjoyed (the only exception being cheese!). I found chocolate, cake, brownies, casseroles, pasta, rice milk, rice, breads, fast food, eating out, and so much more, even a substitute for ice cream! It just took a lot of planning and a bit of ingenuity.

The idea for this guidebook/cookbook came from my husband, who was so supportive of this diet that he ate most of the alternative dishes I prepared, stayed away from most cheese products, and even had rice milk on his cereal. He has always been a supportive eater, and because I love to cook and bake, we make a great combination. We both thought it would have been so much easier if there were some guidelines somewhere on how to survive on this diet. There were no tools, no recipes, no cookbooks, no product guidelines—just a list of ingredients to avoid. Just because you are on a special diet doesn't mean that you stop eating out, stop having to bake for special occasions, stop bringing cookies to school, or stop having holidays. With some help it would have been possible for me to continue breastfeeding, start this diet and survive. So, with much encouragement from my husband, I started writing.

The goal of this book is to be of assistance to the woman who is handed a list of ingredients and told "stay on this diet and you can keep breastfeeding" or "simply avoid all milk and soy products." The word "simply" does not apply here. Once you start reading food labels, you will wonder if there is any food that you can eat! The food substitutions guide will give you quick ideas to get you started and then you can expand into other products and recipes at your own pace.

With the website, you can communicate special problems, share ideas, and be updated on new recipes and product information. The best advice I can give in starting the MSPI diet is to always read labels thoroughly and carefully. This piece of advice, taken with all the other information contained in this book, will get you on your way to eating well. The web address will be www.mspiguide com.

This book is not intended to be a nutrition guide. Though I do try and watch fat and calories in my everyday life, I knew that while breastfeeding I could not diet and I certainly could not do without many of my comfort foods. Simply adding the proper amounts of fruits and vegetables helped me keep my nutrition in check and allowed me a little latitude while navigating this diet. Though I used the MSPI diet strictly for a year, I still find myself using rice milk, figuring out what I could use as dairy substitutes. At a time when much is questioned as to what we add to our foods or feed to our animals in order to make their meat and dairy products "better," many people are turning away from animal products, whether dairy or meat, and trying to figure out reasonable alternatives. This guidebook/cookbook will help you avoid dairy and soy products for whatever reason you are doing so.

The Milk Soy Protein Intolerance (MSPI) Guidebook/Cookbook

GUIDEBOOK

Ingredients to Avoid

Milk Products

milk
cream
milk solids
nonfat dry milk
casein/caseinate
whey
milk chocolate (plus most other chocolates)
butter (plus most all margarines)
lactalbumin

Soy Products*

soy flour
soy protein
soy protein isolate
textured vegetable protein
soy beans
soy caseinate

    *soy oil is okay, as is soy lecithin; they are fats.

Food Substitutions

While there is much it seems that you cannot eat on this diet, there are many things out there that you can use as substitutions. You simply must know where to look. This section will go through each food group and give useful food substitutions, where they exist, for the foods you are giving up. If you get home from shopping and notice that you bought a product that contains one of the 'forbidden' ingredients, take it back. This means you must keep your receipts! The stores I shopped at were very accommodating in refunding money or exchanging products for me when I explained the problem.

IMPORTANT—YOU MUST ALWAYS READ LABELS CAREFULLY. Products may change and it is easy to miss ingredients that should be avoided.

Dairy—there are not any dairy products that are suitable on this diet, because they all contain milk protein, but there are some acceptable alternatives.

Milk—rice milk, almond milk, oat milk.

Rice milk—is available in nearly every grocery store in the health or diet section, for this reason I use rice milk in mostly all recipes. It comes ready to serve or in powdered varieties. It is available enriched, with added calcium, vitamins A and D, and phosphorus. It comes in three flavors: original, vanilla, and chocolate, and some companies sell carob flavor as well.

Almond milk—is available in enriched as well and is available in original and chocolate. It is not stocked in many grocery chains, but it may be ordered through health food stores and is available over the internet.

Oat milk—again available in original, vanilla and chocolate, but it is not as readily available as rice milk is.

Cream/Creamer—there is no a substitute for heavy cream; however, for coffee creamers the rice, almond, and oat milk varieties work quite well. I enjoyed the vanilla-flavored rice milk in my coffee. It certainly lacks the body of cream/milk of other "non-dairy" creamers, but is a good substitute. Beware of "non-dairy" or "lactose-free" creamers, whether liquid or powdered; they often contain soy protein (if they are truly "non-dairy") and also often contain caseinate.

Butter—Fleischmann's unsalted stick margarine, or lowfat sticks or spread were the only substitutes I found. The unsalted sticks are great for baking and cooking, and the lowfat spread is good as a spread for bread and toast. Mazola's unsalted sticks are without milk or soy protein as well. Also check at your local natural foods store; they may have some natural brands that are MSP free.

Crisco—regular or butter flavor, is also useful for baking. You should use a little less Crisco than the of amount butter or margarine that is called for.

Cheese—there is really no substitute for cheese. Although there are many 'rice cheese' products available, they contain caseinate, which is derived from milk, and so they must also be avoided.

***What about goat's milk? Though goat's milk used to be used for many babies (I was one!) who had digestive disturbances that could not be diagnosed and some babies tolerated it, the protein in cow's milk and goat's milk are very similar, so it is not generally recommended as an alternative.

Sour cream—no substitute. I tried to sour rice milk, but it did not work. Again, even "non-dairy" or "lactose-free" sour cream most likely contains either caseinate, whey, or soy protein. (If you use sour cream in Mexican cooking, try substituting guacamole instead; see recipe page 30).

Eggs—eggs are not a dairy product (though they are often referred to as dairy); you may eat eggs and also most egg substitutes.

Spreads/Fats

Oil—nearly any oil may be used. Read labels carefully on flavored oils; some have added milk products to imitate a "buttery" taste.

Peanut Butter—many popular commercial brands of peanut butter contain soy protein. Try a "natural" peanut butter, or your grocery chain's brand. Albertson's brand of creamy and chunky peanut butters do not contain any soy protein as of this writing.

Mayonnaise—Regular or lite varieties of mayonnaise should be okay. In all my checks of both popular and food chain varieties, I failed to find one that listed either milk or soy products.

Mustard—most varieties are acceptable.

Brown Sauces—such as soy, tamari, Worcestershire, hoisin and brown sauce: these all contain soy. If it is brown in color, it mostly likely contains soy, so read the label carefully.

Ketchup, Barbeque sauces—most varieties are acceptable.

Salsa and Picante Sauces—most are acceptable.

Salad Dressings—look for non-creamy varieties here, such as Italian, or vinaigrettes. You must be careful to check for parmesan cheese in some Italian brands. Kraft's Good Seasons Italian, Zesty Italian, and Herb Garlic powdered dressing mixes are milk/soy protein-free.

Hummus—Great spread on breads, for sandwiches or used as a dip. You can find hummus in many flavors in the gourmet or cheese section of most stores. Athenos® is an excellent brand, as is Melissa's®. You must have to be careful to avoid those with cheese (such as feta, or parmesan).

Dips—most commercially packaged dips contain milk products, such as sour cream, milk or whey. Hummus, salsa, bean and guacamole dips are good substitutes for the creamy craving. Guacamole is often best made from scratch as prepackaged varieties can contain milk products for added creaminess (see "Guacamole" recipe, page 30).

Snacks/Desserts

Crackers—There are a few popular brands of crackers that at this printing do not contain any forbidden products. Nabisco's Triscuits, and Wheat Thins, and Carr's Water Crackers are a few. Some brands of crackers may contain whey, cheese, or casein. Pretzels, popcorn, and saltines are often okay. Potato and corn chips are mostly all free of dairy and soy also. Be careful to avoid "flavored" varieties of chips, popcorn, or pretzels; many of the flavorings contain cheese, or whey as an emulsifier.

Cookies—it is hard to find a commercial brand or bakery cookie that is acceptable on this diet, though there are a few. I found the best alternative was to make my own. Like snack crackers, many cookies contain milk products, such as whey, butter fat, casein, and nonfat dry milk.

Chocolate—there are a few brands of semi-sweet chocolate that are acceptable; they are: Ghiradelli semi-sweet chocolate bars and chips, and Newmann's Own semi-sweet chocolate bars (available ones: in regular, espresso, and sweet orange), Guittard semi-sweet chocolate and chocolate chips, and Cloud Nine semi-sweet chocolate and chocolate chips. Don't be fooled by ingredient names, such as cocoa butter: it contains no butter, rather it refers to the 'meat' of the cocoa bean. Soy lecithin is also acceptable, it is a fat, not a protein.

Candy—Most chewy, gummie fruit candies are okay, as are hard candies, except those that contain caramel or chocolate. Caramel flavoring may also contain milk products.

Candy Bars—could not find any acceptable widely commercial brands.

Cakes—you will not be able to eat desserts out at a restaurant or bakery, but you can make cakes and brownies at home that are okay to eat. If you do not have time for the scratch cake recipes found in the cookbook section, many of Duncan Hines's brand cake and brownie mixes are without milk or soy protein. If you write, or call Duncan Hines, they will send you a listing of all their mixes that are dairy/soy protein-free (their address, and phone number are listed in the "Manufacturers" listings). Some of their ready-made frostings are also dairy-free.

Other—plain rice krispy bars are okay (including those manufactured by Kellogg's). Marshmallows and marshmallow cremes are generally okay.

Ice cream and other **frozen desserts**—Yes, as you might have guessed, ice cream is out, but there are some frozen dessert substitutes. Imagine Foods makes a variety of frozen desserts, including 'rice cream,' Dream Bars and Dream Pies. They come in many flavors and are excellent.

Breakfast

Cereals—many of the popular commercial cereals are okay, but read labels carefully. Watch out for single-serving packaged hot-cereal varieties; many contain milk products.

Breakfast Bars—some of Kellogg's Pop-Tart flavors are okay, but nearly all other brands contain milk products in the breading base.

Pancakes/Waffles—whether a packaged mix or frozen variety, most all contain milk and soy products. Much safer to make your own.

Bagels—many franchise bakeries, such as Bruegger's, make several varieties of bagels without milk and/or soy. Watch for the added ingredients in bagels such as "jalapeno cheddar."

Muffins, sweetrolls and **doughnuts**—bad news here: most all commercial brands (including Krispy Kreme) contain nonfat dry milk and possibly other milk and/or soy ingredients. One commercial brand of frozen dough and sweet rolls that I found which is free of milk and soy in many products is Rhodes. As of this printing, their bread dough, sweet dough, cinnamon and orange rolls are free of milk and soy. However, the frosting included with the packaged rolls does contain milk products, so you must make your own.

Other Carbohydrates

Pasta—most all varieties of fresh or dried pasta are okay to use. Boxed pasta mixes with sauces will generally contain milk and/or soy products.

Rice—like pasta, dry rice, steamed or cooked in water, is fine. Many boxed mixes, however, will contain milk and/or soy. Read all labels carefully.

Breads—commercially baked breads and dough products can be tricky. The majority of the breads on the market will contain nonfat dry milk, whey, milk solids, and/or soy flour, and possibly some other milk/soy products. Look for French or Italian breads; go to a bakery and check out their selection. Many grocery chains will bake fresh French or Italian breads that do not contain milk or soy. Go to a bread bakery, such as Great Harvest; many of their breads are suitable as well. Look for kosher or pareve symbols on bread wrappers, such as Rotella, which makes many varieties of bread and rolls that are without milk and soy.

***Watch out for breadings. Nearly all breadings for fried chicken, nuggets, fried or baked fish, and more contain milk and/or soy. Also, bread crumbs that may be used as filler in meatballs, meatloaf, and burgers often contain dry milk, whey, and even some soy proteins.

Beverages

Juices are okay. Look for the juices that contain added calcium for an extra boost (you will need to take a calcium supplement while on this diet). Check with your doctor or dietitian, but most recommend 1200mg calcium per day while pregnant or breastfeeding). Pure vegetable juices are excellent as well. Go to your local juice bar for a treat; just watch for added yogurt, milk, or soy.

Hot drinks such as coffee, tea and chai are okay as long as there is no added milk. You can use the packaged Chai (concentrate) and add your own rice milk; see "Beverages" for recipes. Do be careful of instant flavored coffees, lattés, cappucinos, and teas, they most often will contain milk products. Most instant hot cocoa varieties contain milk products as well.

Soups—watch out for soy protein in most commercial brand soups. Swanson's Natural Goodness brand chicken broth is the only brand I found that did not contain soy protein. Check labels carefully.

Fruits and Vegetables

Fruits—fresh fruits are always great to eat and good for you too! Dried fruits are also an excellent source of vitamins and fiber. Keep some frozen fruits on hand for rice milk shakes. Slice and freeze ripe bananas and use in shakes.

Vegetables—fresh vegetables, like fruits, are very good for you. Keep cut-up carrots and other vegetables handy for snacking. Watch out for sauces on frozen vegetables. The labeling will give you clues, like "buttery" or "light" sauce; then, as always, read the label carefully.

Protein

Meats/Fish—all fresh and frozen plain meats and fish are okay. Watch out for breaded meats and fish; the breading will usually contain milk and/or soy. There is often added soy protein in processed packaged meats, such as pre-made hamburgers, and meatballs and in some varieties of reduced-fat hot dogs, and other meats. There is also soy protein in most hamburger substitutes, such as Gardenburgers® or Boca Burgers®.

Beans—beans are an excellent source of protein and are used throughout this cookbook in a variety of recipes. As with many foods that are gaseous, beans may cause your baby some distress. If you think they are a source of upset to your baby, simply eliminate them for a period to see if the fussiness, gasiness subsides.

**If you are vegetarian, please consult a dietitian to help with planning your diet so you get enough protein. I prefer not to eat a large amount of meat in my diet, and I have been a pure vegetarian; however, I found that during pregnancy I had to add meat for the protein I needed.

A word about kosher/pareve symbols: items that are labeled pareve or parve do not contain any animal products, so, there will be no milk products in these items. A certified Kosher symbol (the symbol is an encircled 'K') means when used on meat items that the product was not made on machinery or with cooking utensils that products containing animal products were made on or with. You will see both the kosher and pareve symbol on Fleischmann's unsalted margarine and on many packages of rotella bread. I used these symbols to help me pick out dairy-free foods, but I checked the labels as well.

Manufacturer/Product Listings

Imagine Foods®—line of rice milk products. Includes regular and enriched rice milks in 4 flavors, frozen deserts, rice milk ice milk in many flavors, puddings, soups and broths. These are excellent products.

Fantastic Foods®—convenient cereals, meals and soups in a microwaveable cup. Other products include pasta and rice mixes. Not all are milk/soy protein free, so read labels carefully.

Nile Spice®—many mixes are milk/soy protein free and are excellent: falafel mix, rice and couscous mixes.

Near East®—pasta and rice mixes; many are milk/soy protein free.

Fleischmann's®—margarine unsalted and lowfat magarines are available in sticks and tub forms. The unsalted sticks are best for baking.

Harmony Farms®—Rice milk, available in 3 flavors, enriched and regular.

Newman's Own Organic Foods®—semi-sweet chocolate bars in plain, sweet orange and espresso.

Albertson's®—nationwide grocery chain with many items that are milk/soy free, including: many fresh-baked breads and rolls, and Albertson's® brand peanut butter. Most stores carry rice milk products and are terrific about ordering specialty items for you.

Great Harvest Bread Company®—nationwide chain of bread bakeries. Old-Fashioned White, Honeywheat and Challah are some of the varieties of bread and rolls that are milk/soy protein-free.

Duncan Hines®—cake, brownie, cookie and muffin mixes that are milk/soy-free. Write to them for a list of their mixes that are milk/soy free.

Atheno's®—packaged hummus dips in a variety of flavors, a few contain milk/cheese. These are good used as dips or spreads.

Ghirardelli®—semi-sweet chocolate bars and chips for eating or baking.

Swanson's Natural Goodness broth®—the only pure chicken broth without added soy protein.

Dr. McDougall's Smart Cup™ meals—soups, pasta, rice and cereals. All are vegetarian, and many are milk/soy protein-free. Very fast and convenient as well.

Riceness®—powdered rice milk, comes in regular and vanilla flavors. Great for traveling, because it can be mixed in smaller quantities.

Better Than Milk®—powdered rice milk, come in original and vanilla flavors and also 'lite,' which has no fat. Again, great for traveling.

Rotella's Italian Bakery®—breads, rolls and buns. All bread products are milk free and certified kosher. Must watch out for soy flour in some breads.

Pacific Foods®—non-dairy beverages (rice, oat and almond milks), organic fruit and vegetable juices, vegetable and chicken broths. Website offers a product locator service.

Guittard®—semi-sweet chocolate chips that are milk and soy protein free.

Ah!laska Products, Inc.®—dairy-free cocoa mixes, cocoa and chocolate syrup. A fabulous Web site! Certified organic and kosher. Sourdough bakery items to order also.

Cloud Nine, Inc.®—semi-sweet and dark chocolates and chocolate bars; 10 percent of their profits go to conserve the rainforest and they use cane juice to sweeten the chocolate. Made from 100 percent organic African cocoa beans. In addition, Cloud Nine chocolates are distributed by Inspired Foods; they also sell many other brands of all natural and organic foods.

Casbah®—natural Middle Eastern food mixes; tahini dressing, tabouli, pilafs, couscous, falafel and more.

Manufacturers' Addresses, Phone and Website Listings:

Imagine Foods, Inc.

350 Cambridge Ave., Suite 350
Palo Alto, CA 94306
info@imaginefoods.com
www.imaginefoods.com
1-800-333-6339

Fleischmann's

Distributed by Beatrice Foods
Indianapolis, IN 46268
1-800-988-7808

Fantastic Foods, Inc.

Petaluma, CA 94954

Dr. McDougall's

101 Utah Avenue
So. San Francisco, CA 94080
drmcdougall@rightfoods.com
www.rightfoods.com
1-650-635-6040

Swanson Natural Goodness Broth

Distributed by Campbell Soup
Company
Camden, NJ 08103-1701
1-800-44-broth

Ghirardelli Chocolate Company

1111 139th Avenue
San Leandro, CA 94578-2631

Near East Food Products

P.O. Box 049006
Chicago, IL 60604-9006
1-800-822-7423

Duncan Hines

Distributed by Aurora Foods, Inc.
Columbus, OH 43235
1-800-254-3768
www.aurorafoods.com

Riceness

Made by Fearn Natural Foods
6425 West Executive Drive
Mequon, WI 53092

Harmony Farms

Distributed by American Natural
    Snacks
P.O. Box 1067
St. Augustone, FL 32085-1067

Athenos

Mediterranean Spreads,
    distributed by
    Churny Company, Inc.
Weyauwega, WI 54983
1-800-343-1976

Better Than Milk

Fuller Life Inc.
1628 Robert C. Jackson Dr.
Maryville, TN 37801
1-800-227-2320
www.betterthanmilk.com

Rotella's Italian Bakery, Inc.

6949 South 108th Street
Omaha, NE 68128
1-800-759-0360
www.rotellas/bakery.com

**Great Harvest Bread
Company**

28 South Montana
Dillon, MT 59725
1-800-442-0424
www.greatharvest.com

Pacific Foods, Inc.

19480 SW 97th Avenue
Tualatin, OR 97062
1-503-692-9666
pfo@pacificfoods.com
www.pacificfoods.com

**Guittard Chocolate
Company**

10 Guittard Road
Burlingame, CA 94011-4308
1-800-468-2462
Fax: 1-650-692-2761
www.guittard.com

Ah!laska Products, Inc.

P.O. Box 940
Homer, AK 99603
907-235-2673
www.ahlaska.com

Cloud Nine, Inc.

Inspired Natural Foods
300 Observer Highway
Hoboken, N.J. 07030
201-216-0382
www.nspiredfoods.com

Casbah

Sahara Natural Foods, Inc.
P.O. Box 11844
Berkeley, CA 94704

On-Line Shopping

www.wholefoods.com—at Wholefoods you can buy bulk rice milk, cereals, flours, grains, spices, Newman's Own chocolate, and much more.

www.bpco-op.com—Blooming Prairie Co-op. Many natural foods in bulk, check out how to be a member.

www.albertsons.com—to find grocery stores near you, product information and online shopping.

www.pacificfoods.com—to order bulk rice milk, broth, and other items.

www.kingsmillfoods.com—allergy sensitive foods. Rice breads, rice baking mixes. Cookies and cookie base.

Cyber-Sources

www.skyisland.com/online resources—Information on food allergies and intolerances, online cookbook and substitutions page.

www.foodallergy.com—information on food allergies, cookbooks and nutrition.

www.cyberdiet.com—more general information on diet, nutrition, and exercise.

www.wholehealthmd.com—general information on health, diet, and natural healing. Includes an online library, shopping and recipes.

www.babymilk.com—facts on infant nutrition, breastfeeding, and more.

www.mothers.org—information on mothering, products, foods, and much more.

www.lactose.net—information about lactose intolerance and related topics.

www.montanarob.homestead.com—home of the "No Moo" cookbook and other information on milk allergies and intolerance.

www.geocities.com/hotspring/4620/.—no nonsense information on soy allergies.

Special Circumstances

Eating Out . . .

My best advice on eating out is to call ahead. I would first explain my special circumstances and then ask if there were items on their menu that might be milk/soy protein free. To my surprise in most every restaurant I called there was someone who would take the time to go through the menu with me and even read ingredients off labels for me; in fact I often talked directly to the chef. One of my older son's favorite eateries was a local burger restaurant; they took the time to tell me about the meat (no fillers in the hamburger) and read through the label on the hamburger buns, which let me know that I could eat the burgers, but not the buns. Which brings me to another piece of advice. . . .

Bring items with you that you know are milk/soy protein free. I always brought my own hamburger buns to the aforementioned restaurant, and if I was going to have salad, I brought my own salad dressing. To my surprise, no one ever said a word about it. I think I explained the situation many times because of my own awkwardness, but no one ever questioned me. Items that I frequently brought out with me were: margarine, buns, bread, salad dressings, and maybe a cookie, or a piece of chocolate if I knew everyone else would be having dessert. That way, I never had to feel left out.

In choosing menu items, I always figured that grilled meat was pretty safe, so long as they didn't baste it in butter or marinade containing soy sauce. Most salads were okay also, as long as they were made without cheese, croutons, and served with the dressing on the side. I would always let my waiter know what my needs were as well; that way they could help guide me in my choices. Dessert was always forbidden, unless I made it.

If you are really lucky, your town has a kosher deli! What a goldmine! There you can be assured that no bread will contain milk products, because kosher law forbids the mixing of milk products with meat. And you can, for the same reason, trust the soups. Just make sure bread and soups do not contain any soy flour or soy protein.

Health food, or "natural food" restaurants are also terrific!

When invited out for dinner . . .

Again, call ahead. I would always call the host or hostess a few days before the date, explain my special circumstances, and ask about the menu. I never wanted anyone to feel that they had to change the menu for me, but only that it would help me to know what was planned in advance so I could bring anything I needed to supplement my meal. Then, I would always ask to bring something—dessert was my usual offering—that way I knew I could at least indulge in dessert with everyone else!

Outdoor potluck dinners on the grill were particularly easy; you could bring your own meat, margarine for a baked potato, salad dressing and dessert. One time when we were invited out, the hostess was planning lasagna, salad, and vegetables. I brought a grilled chicken breast, my own dressing, and had it over salad, and of course, I offered to bring some dessert so I could partake as well. It all worked out perfectly.

Fast Food . . .

Always call the 1-800 numbers each of the fast food, or chain restaurants (or for that matter food manufacturers) make available. You will speak with someone who usually has nutritional information at his or her fingertips. For instance, one of my favorite fast foods is a bean burrito at Taco Bell. I called Taco Bell's 1-800 number, and they were able to go through the ingredients on their flour tortillas (which contain no milk/soy protein), their guacamole (again, milk/soy protein-free), and their refried beans (which are also milk/soy protein-free). So, I could have a bean burrito, minus the cheese (which I usually replaced with lettuce and tomato, or guacamole), and a seven-layer burrito, minus the cheese and sour cream. They were terrific, and it gave me a fast food alternative that I really liked. Choose the fast food restaurant that you enjoy most and call them; explore the options that are available to you!

You do become the 'food police' when on this diet, knowing that if you mess up, your baby pays for it. So you will become very suspicious, but don't feel bad about asking questions. Most people are more than willing to help you wade your way through a pile of ingredients!

22

COOKBOOK

Beverages

Banana Shake

8 ounces enriched vanilla rice milk, chilled

1 banana, sliced (may be fresh or frozen)
1/4 cup crushed ice

Put all ingredients into blender and blend until smooth. Serve immediately.

Chocolate-Banana Shake

8 ounces enriched chocolate rice milk, chilled
1 banana, sliced (fresh or frozen)
1 teaspoon vanilla flavoring (or

try almond for a different taste)
1 tablespoon Ah!laska® dairy free cocoa mix
1/4 cup crushed ice

Put all ingredients into blender and blend until smooth. Sweeten to taste. Serve immediately.

Healthy Breakfast Shake

8 ounces enriched rice milk, chilled
1 banana, sliced

1 teaspoon vanilla or almond extract
1 tablespoon wheat germ
1/4 teaspoon cinnamon

Put all ingredients into blender and blend until smooth. Serve immediately.

Tropical Fruit Shake

1 cup vanilla Rice Dream frozen
    dessert
1/3 cup pineapple juice

1/4 cup orange juice
1 ripe banana, sliced

Put all ingredients into blender and blend until smooth. Serve immediately.

Berry Smoothie

1/2 cup frozen strawberries
1/4 cup frozen blueberries
1/4 cup frozen raspberries

1 cup enriched vanilla rice milk,
    chilled

Place all ingredients into blender and purée until smooth. Sweeten to taste. Serve immediately.

Banana-Strawberry Shake

1/2 cup frozen strawberries
1 ripe banana, sliced

1 cup enriched rice milk, chilled

Place all ingredients into blender and blend until smooth. Sweeten to taste. Serve immediately.

Chocolate Raspberry Shake

1/2 cup frozen raspberries
1 cup enriched chocolate rice
    milk, chilled

1 teaspoon vanilla extract
1 tablespoon Ah!laska® dairy
    free cocoa mix

Place all ingredients into blender and blend until smooth. Sweeten to taste. Serve immediately.

Peach-Berry Shake

1/2 cup frozen peaches
1/2 cup frozen raspberries

1 cup enriched vanilla rice milk,
chilled

Place all ingredients into blender and blend until smooth. Sweeten to taste. Serve immediately.

Orange Banana Fiber Shake

1 ripe banana, frozen and sliced
4-5 orange-flavored prunes,
chopped

1/2 cup orange juice
1 cup enriched vanilla rice milk,
chilled

Place all ingredients into blender and blend until smooth. Serve immediately.

**Tips for shakes: Take overripe bananas and slice, wrap in plastic and freeze. Using frozen bananas helps thicken up the shake. If bananas are fresh, may use 1/4 cup crushed ice to thicken. Add 1 tablespoon bran or wheat germ to boost the fiber in your shake. Some are not terribly sweet, so you may want to add 1 packet of Equal or sugar to desired sweetness.

Hot Beverages

Chai

1 cup chai concentrate (available in most coffee houses and some grocery stores)

1 cup enriched rice milk (you may add more rice milk to taste)

Heat together in microwave-safe mug, about 2 to 3 minutes. Stir and serve.

Vanilla Chai

1 cup chai concentrate

1 cup, or more, enriched vanilla rice milk

Heat altogether in a microwave-safe mug, about 2 to 3 minutes. Stir and serve.

Chocolate Chai

1 cup chai concentrate
1 cup enriched chocolate rice milk

1 tablespoon Ah!laska® cocoa mix

Heat together in a microwave-safe mug, about 2 to 3 minutes. Stir and serve.

Hot Cocoa

1/3 cup cocoa powder
1/2 cup granulated sugar

4 cups enriched vanilla rice milk

Stir ingredients together in a medium saucepan over medium heat. Heat thoroughly while stirring, but do not allow to boil. Makes 4 one-cup servings or 2 larger servings. Marshmallows are optional!

Hot Cocoa Ah!laska Style

2 cups enriched rice milk

4 rounded teaspoons Ah!laska brand dairy-free cocoa mix

First, heat milk in a microwave safe container. Stir in cocoa mix and serve.
Great as a cold drink as well!

Café Latte

1/2 cup *strong* coffee
1 cup enriched rice milk
1-2 ounces flavored coffee syrup

(vanilla, almond, Irish creme, etc.)

Heat all coffee and rice milk together in a microwave-safe mug, about 2 to 3 minutes. Stir in syrup and serve.

Appetizers

Black Bean Rollups

4 ten-inch flour tortillas
1 fifteen-ounce can black beans, drained
1/4 cup enriched rice milk
2 green onions, chopped

1/8 cup cilantro, minced
1/2 cup yellow pepper, chopped
1/4 cup green olives, chopped
1/2 teaspoon garlic salt

Purée beans in a food processor or blender. Stir in rice milk, onion, cilantro, and garlic salt. Spread bean mixture evenly over 4 tortillas. Top with even amounts of yellow pepper and green olives. Roll tortilla up tightly and wrap. Chill in refrigerator 1-2 hours. Cut into 3/4-inch slices to serve. Serve with salsa, and/or guacamole (next recipe).

Guacamole

3 ripe avocados, peeled and mashed
1 teaspoon onion powder
1 teaspoon garlic salt

1 cup Roma tomatoes, diced
1 tablespoon lime juice

Mix seasoning, tomatoes, and lime juice into avocado and stir well. Refrigerate before serving. Serve with tortilla chips, or crackers. Great with burritos and other Mexican fare.

Chile Lime Hummus

2 fifteen-ounce cans garbanzo
    beans, drained
1/4 cup tahini (sesame seed paste)
1/3 cup lime juice

2 tablespoons cider vinegar
1 tablespoon minced garlic
1 teaspoon chile powder
1 teaspoon seasoning salt
pinch cayenne pepper

Combine all ingredients in food processor and blend until smooth. Use as a spread on bread, pita, crackers, or tortillas.

Stuffed Mushrooms

20-24 mushrooms, washed, stems removed, reserved and chopped
2 tablespoons olive oil
1 teaspoon garlic, minced
2/3 cup red bell pepper, diced
2 green onions, chopped
1 & 1/2 tablespoons parsley, minced
1/2 cup bread crumbs
1/2 teaspoon chile powder
1 & 1/2 teaspoons salt
all-vegetable cooking spray

In a medium skillet, combine olive oil and garlic. Heat over medium heat until garlic is light golden brown. Sauté together chopped mushroom stems, bell pepper, onion until slightly tender, 2 to 3 minutes. Add parsley and bread crumbs and sauté 1 to 2 more minutes. Remove from heat, add chile powder and salt. Set aside and cool.

Spray a large baking dish with cooking spray. Spoon stuffing into the mushroom caps, distribute evenly. Place stuffed mushroom caps in baking dish. At this point, mushroom caps may be covered and refrigerated for several hours. When ready to serve, preheat oven to 425 degrees. Place baking dish in upper third of oven and bake 10 to 15 minutes until bubbly and tender.

Eggplant and Garlic Spread

1 large eggplant
4 garlic cloves, peeled
2 tablespoons olive oil
juice of 1/4 lemon
1 teaspoon oregano flakes
1/2 teaspoon cumin powder
1 teaspoon salt
all-vegetable cooking spray

Preheat oven to 450 degrees. Cut eggplant in half and place in baking dish sprayed with cooking spray, cut side down. Slip 2 garlic cloves under each eggplant half, and bake for 1 hour, or until tender. Cool.

Scrape pulp from eggplant halves, drain in colander, until excess moisture is gone. Place eggplant pulp, garlic, oil, lemon juice, oregano and seasoning in food processor. Process until smooth. May use more salt and pepper to taste. Use as a spread with crackers, vegetables, bread or pita.

Pesto Pizza

1 dough recipe from page 46   1 package sun-dried tomatoes
1 pesto recipe from page 55

Roll, or press out dough into a large round. Poke holes in top of dough with a fork. Spread pesto gently over top of dough, then add sun-dried tomatoes evenly over surface. Bake at 400 degrees for 10 to 15 minutes, until dough is puffed and golden brown. Keep an eye on this during baking so that sun-dried tomatoes do not burn.

Another way to keep sun-dried tomatoes from burning is to soak them in one cup of warm water a half hour before using them.

Salads

Black Bean and Rice Salad

(*serves 8*)
2 & 1/2 cups chicken broth
1 & 1/4 cups white rice (long
    grain)
1 fifteen-ounce can black beans,
    rinsed and drained
1 pound plum tomatoes, seeded
    and chopped (about 6)
1/2 cup green bell pepper,
    chopped
1/2 cup yellow bell pepper,
    chopped
1 cup chopped onion (Vidalia, or
    sweet variety)
1/4 cup vinegar
2 tablespoons olive oil
juice of 1 lime
1 tablespoon chopped garlic
1 tablespoon chopped cilantro

Bring chicken broth to boil in a large saucepan; add rice, cover pan, and simmer over reduced heat until tender (about 20 minutes). Transfer to a large bowl and cool to room temperature.

Add black beans, tomato, peppers and onion to rice, and mix well. In a separate small bowl, whisk remainder of the ingredients together. Pour dressing over salad and toss. Add salt and pepper to taste. Serve at room temperature.

White Bean Salad

(*serves 8*)
2 sixteen-ounce cans great north-
    ern beans, rinsed and
    drained
1 & 1/2 cup plum tomatoes,
    chopped
1/2 cup sweet onion, chopped
2 tablespoons olive oil
1 clove garlic, chopped
1/4 cup parsley, chopped
juice of 1/2 lemon
1/4 cup white vinegar

Heat 1 tablespoon olive oil over medium-high heat and sauté garlic till just browned. Remove from heat. Add garlic to remaining tablespoon olive oil, whisk in parsley, lemon juice, and vinegar until blended.

In a large bowl, combine beans, tomatoes and onion. Pour dressing over top and toss. Chill and then serve.

Sautéed Cajun Salad

8 cups mixed spring greens
spicy Italian salad dressing
2 tablespoons olive oil
1 pound (16 ounces) cooked medium shrimp
1 small package pre-sliced turkey pepperoni
1 cup onion, coarsely chopped
1 red bell pepper, coarsely chopped
2 garlic cloves, chopped
1 cup canned black beans, rinsed and drained
1-2 tablespoons Cajun seasoning, to taste
2 Granny Smith apples, sliced in wedges (about 8 per apple), not peeled

Divide spring greens evenly among serving plates.

Heat oil in a large skillet over medium heat. Add onion, red pepper and garlic, and sauté 2-3 minutes. Without reducing heat, add shrimp and pepperoni and cook an additional 5 minutes while stirring constantly (stir-fry style). Reduce heat to medium and add black beans and cajun spice, stirring well and frequently. Add apples and cook another 1-2 minutes until heated.

Drizzle Italian salad dressing over spring greens and then divide sautéed mixture evenly and spoon over prepared salad. Serve while still warm. Serves 4.

Tabbouleh

3 cups fresh parsley, minced
1/3 cup fresh mint leaves, minced
2 cups cucumber, seeded and chopped
2 cups Roma tomatoes, seeded and chopped
1/2 cup green onions, chopped
1 four-ounce can chopped black olives
1 & 1/2 cups bulgur or cracked wheat, uncooked
2 tablespoons olive oil
juice of 1 lemon
1 teaspoon garlic salt

Combine all ingredients in a large bowl and toss. Refrigerate for several hours, or overnight to marinate. Serves 4-6.

Waldorf Chicken Salad

(*serves 4-6*)

2-3 cooked large chicken breasts
(boiled or grilled), cut into
chunks
1 cup brown rice, cooked (may use
regular or minute variety)
1 cup seedless red grapes

1 Granny Smith apple, diced
1 cup diced celery
1/3 cup reduced fat mayonnaise
1/4 teaspoon ground ginger
1/2 teaspoon ground cinnamon
juice from 1/2 lemon

Squeeze lemon over diced apple and mix. Combine apple with other ingredients, stirring in mayonnaise and spices until well blended. Serve over fresh lettuce leaves and garnish with fruit.

Raspberry Spinach Salad

8 cups spinach, rinsed and torn
into bite-size pieces
1 cup raspberries
3 kiwis, peeled and sliced
3/4 cup chopped macadamia nuts

Dressing:
2 tablespoons raspberry vinegar
2 tablespoons raspberry jam
1 tablespoon sugar
1/3 cup canola oil

Assemble salad ingredients in large bowl. Mix dressing until well blended. Drizzle dressing on salad and toss. Serves 6.

Asparagus Salad

2 small cans mandarin oranges,
drain and reserve 2 tablespoons juice
1 tablespoon canola oil
6 cups asparagus, cut in 2-inch
pieces (about 2 lbs.)

1 clove garlic, chopped
1/2 cup sliced almonds
1/2 teaspoon dark sesame oil
2 tablespoons sesame seeds,
toasted
romaine or greenleaf lettuce leaves

Heat canola oil in a skillet over medium heat. Add asparagus, garlic and almonds, and sauté about 5 minutes. Remove from pan. Pour sesame oil over asparagus and mix well. Cool to room temperature. Stir in sesame seeds, juice and oranges. Serve on lettuce leaves. Serves 6 to 8. (Excellent as a side dish as well, just leave off the lettuce leaves.)

Mandarin Salad

6 cups salad greens
1/2 cup sliced almonds
1 cup chopped celery
1 green onion, chopped
1 eleven-ounce can mandarin or-
    anges, drained (reserve 1 ta-
    blespoon juice for dressing)

Dressing:
1/4 cup canola oil
2 tablespoons sugar
2 tablespoons rice vinegar
1/2 teaspoon salt
1 tablespoon chopped parsley

Mix salad greens, almonds, celery, green onion and oranges together. In a separate small bowl, whisk together dressing ingredients until well blended. Pour dressing over salad and toss to coat. Serves 4-6.

Palm Salad

12 cups mixed salad greens
1 fourteen-ounce can hearts of
    palm, chopped
1 four-ounce can of sliced black
    olives
2 cups grape or cherry tomatoes,
    rinsed and halved

Dressing:
1/3 cup olive oil
3 tablespoons red wine vinegar
1/2 teaspoon salt
1/4 teaspoon oregano
1 teaspoon minced garlic

Toss salad ingredients together in a large bowl. Combine dressing ingredients and whisk, or shake to blend. Drizzle dressing over salad and toss. Serves 8.

Shrimp Tostada Salad

1 pound medium-cooked shrimp,
    tails removed
1 tablespoon olive oil
1 teaspoon sesame oil
1 teaspoon garlic, minced
1 teaspoon cumin
1 teaspoon jalapeno chiles,
    minced
1 fifteen-ounce can black beans,
    drained and rinsed
2 & 1/2 cups Roma tomatoes,
    chopped
2 ears fresh corn, kernels cut
    from cobs
1 cup green onion, chopped
1/2 cup cilantro, chopped
1 head iceberg lettuce, shredded

Dressing:
1/4 cup canola oil
1/2 cup lime juice with pulp
1 tablespoon white vinegar
1 teaspoon ground cumin
1/2 teaspoon salt
1/2 teaspoon garlic, minced
tortilla chips and cilantro for garnish

Heat olive and sesame oil in a large skillet over medium-high heat. Add shrimp, garlic, cumin, jalapeno and corn, and sauté until warmed thoroughly, about 5 to 7 minutes. Remove from heat. When mixture is cool, stir in black beans, tomato, green onion and cilantro.

Blend dressing ingredients together in a small bowl. Arrange lettuce on plates, with tortilla chips around edges. Pour dressing over shrimp/black bean mixture and toss to coat. Spoon evenly over lettuce on plates. Garnish and serve.

Pesto Pasta Salad

1/4 cup pesto (for recipe, see page 55)
8 ounces cooked rotini or cork-
    screw pasta
1 cup broccoli florets
1 cup cherry or grape tomatoes,
    halved

1 jar marinated artichoke hearts,
    drained and quartered
1 four-ounce can sliced black olives
1 four-ounce jar button mush-
    rooms, drained

Mix all ingredients except pesto in large bowl. Stir in pesto and toss to coat. Season to taste with salt and pepper. Chill and serve.

Cabbage Salad

1/2 head green cabbage, sliced
1/2 cup sliced almonds
2 green onions, chopped
2 packages ramen-style noodles,
    crumbled

Dressing:
3 tablespoons canola oil
2 tablespoons sugar
3 tablespoons rice vinegar
2 tablespoons sesame seeds
salt and pepper

Toss first 4 ingredients in a large bowl. Place all dressing ingredients in an airtight container and shake to blend. Pour dressing over salad and toss to coat. Let marinate in refrigerator 2 hours before serving.

Marinated Vegetable Salad

1 bunch broccoli, rinsed and sep-
    arated into florets
1 small head cauliflower, rinsed
    and separated into florets
2 cups cherry or grape tomatoes,
    rinsed and halved

1 four-ounce jar button mush-
    rooms, drained
2 cups carrots, sliced
2 stalks celery, sliced
1 fifteen-ounce can black olives,
    drained
2 cups bottled Italian dressing

Mix all ingredients together in a large bowl. Pour Italian dressing over and toss to coat. Refrigerate and marinate for 2 hours, then serve. Makes a large quantity and keeps for up to a week.

Potato Salad

6 to 8 medium potatoes, cooked
    with skins on and diced
3/4 cup celery, chopped
3 green onions, chopped
2 hard boiled eggs, separate egg
    yolk from whites and re-
    serve, chop egg whites

1/2 cup green olives with pimen-
    tos, sliced
1 tablespoon Dijon-style mustard
1/2 cup lowfat mayonnaise
1/4 cup lemon juice
salt and pepper to taste

Combine potatoes, celery, onion, olives, and egg whites in a large bowl. In a separate small bowl, blend or mash egg yolks into mayonnaise and mustard. Stir in lemon juice. Stir dressing into potato mixture. Season with salt and pepper. Chill and serve.

Soups

Vegetarian Chili

2 tablespoons olive oil
1 cup onion, chopped
1/2 cup green pepper, chopped
3 large cloves garlic, minced
2 teaspoons chile powder
1 teaspoon oregano
1 twenty-four ounce can V-8 juice (may use spicy or regular)
1 four-ounce can chopped green chiles
1 sixteen-ounce can kidney beans
1 sixteen-ounce can pinto beans
1 four-ounce can chopped black olives
1/3 cup bulgur wheat

Heat olive oil in a large non-stick saucepan over medium-high heat. Sauté onion and green pepper until tender. Add garlic and sauté 2 additional minutes. Turn off heat and stir in chile powder and oregano. Add V-8 juice and bulgur wheat, and heat to boil. Then reduce heat, cover, and simmer for 20 minutes. Add beans, chiles, and olives and simmer an additional 20 minutes.

White Chili

3 fifteen-ounce cans Great Northern beans, undrained
4 large chicken breasts (boiled or grilled), cut into bite-sized pieces (or 1 rotisserie chicken, skinned and cut into bite-sized pieces)
2 tablespoons olive oil
1 large onion, chopped
3 cloves garlic, chopped
1 teaspoon chile powder
1 teaspoon cumin
2 teaspoons oregano
2 four-ounce cans chopped green chiles
6 cups canned chicken broth

In a large saucepan over medium-high heat, sauté onion and garlic in olive oil until onion is tender. Reduce heat and add green chiles, spices and oregano. Add chicken broth, beans and chicken, and simmer for 20-30 minutes. Salt and pepper to taste.

Chicken Chowder

2 tablespoons olive oil
1 cup chopped onion
1 cup chopped red bell pepper
2 garlic cloves, chopped
5 cups chicken broth
3 cups diced red potatoes
2 1/2 cups whole kernel corn
1 1/2 cups enriched rice milk

1/3 cup all-purpose flour
1 store-bought rotisserie chicken,
    skinned, meat cut off, and
    cubed
salt and pepper to taste
1/2 cup crumbled bacon
1/2 cup sliced green onion

Heat olive oil over medium-high heat in a large saucepan. Sauté onion, red pepper and garlic for 5 minutes, reduce heat and add chicken broth. Add potatoes and simmer 20 minutes or until potatoes are tender, add corn and chicken. In a small bowl, whisk flour and rice milk until well blended, pour into broth while stirring constantly. Simmer soup over medium heat 15-20 minutes or until slightly thickened, stirring frequently. Add salt and pepper to taste. Top with crumbled bacon (turkey or other) and sliced onions, and serve.

Sweet Potato and Apple Soup

1 teaspoon olive oil
1 onion, chopped
3 cloves garlic, chopped
3 cups chicken broth

2 large sweet potatoes, peeled
    and chopped
2 large Granny Smith apples,
    peeled, seeded and chopped
1 & 1/2 cups enriched rice milk
1/2 teaspoon cinnamon

Heat oil in a large saucepan on medium-high heat. Add onion and garlic and sauté until tender, about 5 minutes. Add chicken broth and bring to a boil. Add sweet potatoes and apples to chicken broth, reduce to medium heat, cover and simmer until potatoes and apples are tender; about 25 minutes.

Purée potato and apple mixture until slightly chunky, working in small batches, then return mixture to saucepan. Stir in rice milk and cinnamon. Season with salt and pepper, and serve. Serves 6.

Chicken Noodle Soup

1 rotisserie chicken, skin removed, chicken cut in bite-sized pieces
1 cup celery, chopped
1 cup carrots, chopped
1 cup sliced mushrooms, fresh or canned
1 cup onion, chopped
2 cloves garlic, chopped
2 tablespoons olive oil
1/4 cup parsley (dried or fresh)
1 package frozen egg noodles
6 cups chicken broth
salt and pepper to taste

Heat oil in large saucepan on medium high heat. Add onion, garlic and celery and sauté 5 minutes. Add mushrooms and sauté another 5 minutes. Stir in carrots and parsley. Add chicken broth to mixture and bring to a boil. Stir in egg noodles, cover and simmer on reduced heat until noodles are tender (15-20 minutes). Add chicken and heat thoroughly. Salt and pepper to taste and serve.

Beef Barley Soup

4 tablespoons margarine
1 teaspoon garlic, chopped
1 yellow onion, chopped
1 cup mushrooms, sliced
2 medium carrots, peeled and sliced
1/3 cup parsley, chopped
8 cups beef broth
1 cup barley
salt and pepper to taste

In a large stockpot, melt margarine and then sauté garlic and onion over medium-high heat, about 5 minutes. Add mushrooms and continue to sauté another 5 minutes. Add carrots and parsley and sauté for an additional 5 minutes. Pour beef broth over mixture and heat to a boil. Add barley and reduce heat to simmer. Simmer, while covered, until barley is tender, and stock is slightly reduced, about 45 minutes. Salt and pepper to taste and serve.

Main Courses

Chicken Primavera Fettucine with Lemon Garlic Sauce

10-12 fresh chicken tenders
1 cup julienne sliced carrots
1 cup julienne sliced zucchini
1/2 cup yellow bell pepper, sliced
   thin
1 cup sliced mushrooms
12 ounces spinach fettucine
1 teaspoon seasoning salt
1 tablespoon margarine

cooking spray
Sauce:
2 tablespoons margarine
1 teaspoon minced garlic
1 cup chicken broth
1 cup enriched rice milk
2 tablespoons flour
juice of 1 lemon
1/4 cup chopped parsley

Heat a medium non-stick skillet over medium-high heat. Add chicken tenders, sprinkle over seasoning salt, and sauté until cooked through and lightly browned. Remove chicken and drain on paper towels. Melt 1 tablespoon margarine in skillet and add garlic, sauté over medium high heat until slightly browned. Then add vegetables and mushrooms and stir-fry until slightly tender, about 5 to 6 minutes. Set aside.

Bring water to boil in a large pot. Add pasta when water is boiling and cook to desired tenderness. Drain.

In a medium saucepan, melt margarine. In a separate small bowl, blend flour and rice milk. Add chicken broth and rice milk/flour mixture to the melted margarine and heat over medium high. While stirring constantly, bring mixture to a boil. Boil 1 minute, then remove from heat. Stir in lemon juice and parsley.

In large pot, combine pasta, chicken, vegetables and sauce, and toss to coat. Serve immediately.

Spinach Fettucine with Sun-dried Tomatoes

12 ounces dry spinach fettucine
1 cup chicken broth
1/3 cup enriched rice milk
2 tablespoons flour
1 six-ounce jar marinated artichoke hearts, drained and
marinade reserved
1/2 cup boiling water
1 cup sun-dried tomatoes (dry,
not packed in oil)
2 green onions, chopped
salt and pepper

Boil a large pot of water and cook pasta until tender. Place sun-dried tomatoes in a small bowl and pour in boiling water, let sit while pasta cooks. In a medium saucepan over medium heat, add artichoke marinade and chicken broth. Bring to a boil for 2 to 3 minutes, reduce heat and add rice milk and whisk in flour until smooth. Cook over medium-high heat until sauce begins to boil, while stirring constantly. Remove from heat and set aside.

Drain excess water off tomatoes. Mix tomatoes, artichokes and green onion into sauce and stir over medium heat until heated through. Drain pasta, then return it to large pot, pour sauce over top, and toss. Season with salt and pepper and serve. Yield: 4 servings.

Creamy Chicken Noodle Bake

1 rotisserie chicken, skinned and
cut into bite-sized chunks
2 tablespoons margarine
1 teaspoon garlic, minced
1/2 cup onion, chopped
1 cup zucchini, chopped
1 cup mushrooms, sliced (fresh
or canned)
1/2 cup flour
2 cups enriched rice milk
1 1/2 cups chicken broth
1 teaspoon salt
8 ounces spinach fettucine (or 1/2
regular and 1/2 spinach)
2 tablespoons margarine
1 cup breadcrumbs (Rotella®)
1 teaspoon seasoning salt
all-vegetable cooking spray

In a large saucepan, melt margarine, then sauté garlic, onion, zucchini and mushrooms until slightly tender. Set aside.

Whisk 1 cup rice milk with flour in a medium saucepan, until smooth. Set heat on medium high and add remaining rice milk and chicken broth.

Stir until mixture thickens and just starts to boil, add salt and remove from heat.

Cook fettucine in a large pot of boiling water until just tender. Drain and then return to saucepan. Mix in chicken, onion and zucchini mixture, mushrooms and white sauce. Pour into a 13 x 9-inch casserole dish, coated with cooking spray.

In a small skillet, melt margarine and sauté breadcrumbs for 2 minutes over medium high heat. Stir in seasoning salt. Sprinkle over top of casserole. Bake at 375 degrees, until casserole bubbles and breadcrumbs are golden brown. Let set for 10 to 15 minutes and serve.

Shrimp and Parsley Pasta

1 pound cooked medium shrimp, detailed
12 ounces spaghetti, or linguine pasta
1 fifteen-and-a-half-ounce can chicken broth
1 tablespoon cornstarch
2 tablespoons margarine
1/2 teaspoon chopped garlic
1 tablespoon chopped parsley
juice of 1/2 lemon

Place a large saucepan full of water on high heat. In a large skillet, heat margarine on medium-high heat until melted. Add garlic and sauté until lightly browned. Add shrimp and sauté until heated thoroughly (about 5 minutes), then turn heat to low.

When water is boiling, add pasta and stir. Reduce heat to medium and keep pasta boiling. Combine broth and cornstarch in a small bowl, whisk or blend to mix thoroughly. Then pour broth and cornstarch mixture over the shrimp mixture and increase heat to medium, stirring constantly. Continue stirring mixture over medium-high heat until it thickens, then reduce heat to low. Add lemon juice and parsley.

Check pasta for desired tenderness and drain. Pour pasta into a large (preferably warmed) serving bowl. Pour shrimp mixture over the pasta and toss. Serve immediately. Serves 4-6.

Calzones

Filling:
1 lb fresh lean ground beef
1 twenty-six-ounce jar pasta
    sauce with green and black
    olives
1 fifteen-ounce can artichoke
    hearts, quartered

Dough:
1 cup lukewarm water
1 teaspoon honey or sugar
1 tablespoon active dry yeast
2 & 1/2 cups all-purpose flour,
    plus extra flour for working
    the dough
1/2 teaspoon salt
all-vegetable cooking spray

Mix the water and honey/sugar in a medium mixing bowl. Sprinkle the yeast on top and set aside until bubbles appear on the surface. Mix the flour and salt together in the bowl of a food processor. Gradually drizzle in the yeast mixture while the processor is on. Continue to process until a ball forms. If the dough is too sticky, add a little more flour and process or knead in.

Turn out the ball of dough into a large mixing bowl coated with cooking spray, coat the top of the dough with a thin layer of cooking spray, cover and let rise until doubled in size.

While dough is rising, brown the ground beef in a large skillet, then drain. Add pasta sauce and artichoke hearts, mix well.

Preheat oven to 375 degrees.

Remove dough and place on a floured work surface. Roll out to approximately 1/2 inch thickness. Divide into 4 equal pieces.

Spoon the sauce and ground beef mixture into the center of each piece of dough, about 3/4 to 1 cup in each (you may have some sauce and ground beef mixture left—it's great over pasta!) Fold over the edge of the dough and crimp edges together. Spray top of dough with a light coating of cooking spray.

Bake for 15-20 minutes, or until golden brown. Let set for 5-10 minutes and serve.

Chicken Cacciatore

10 to 12 fresh chicken tenders
1 twenty-six-ounce jar pasta
  sauce with mushrooms and
  black olives
1 fifteen-ounce can artichoke
  hearts, drained and quartered
1 twelve-ounce package pasta,
  spaghetti or rotini
cooking spray

Bring a large saucepan of water to a rapid boil. Add pasta and cook until tender.

Once the water is on for the pasta, sauté chicken in a pan coated with cooking spray, until golden brown and cooked through. Add pasta sauce and artichoke hearts to chicken.

Pour cooked pasta into a 13 x 9-inch pan coated with cooking spray and cover with sauce and chicken mixture. Heat in oven at 300 degrees until warmed through and serve.

Note: this dish may be made as a casserole, as above, or you may arrange the cooked pasta onto plates and spoon the chicken and sauce mixture over top; then serve immediately.

Broccoli Chicken

10-12 chicken tenders
1 teaspoon garlic, minced
2 cups broccoli florets
1 recipe clear chicken gravy (see
  page 53)

In a large skillet, stir-fry chicken and garlic over medium-high heat until cooked through. Add broccoli and stir-fry until it is deep green in color and slightly tender. Reduce heat to low and add clear chicken gravy. Simmer 10 minutes. Serve over steamed rice. Season to taste with salt and pepper.

Lemon Chicken

2 tablespoons margarine
1 tablespoon olive oil
salt and pepper
4 boneless chicken breasts
2 teaspoons garlic, minced

1 cup chicken broth
1/4 cup lemon juice
lemon for garnish
fresh parsley, chopped

In a large skillet with high sides, melt margarine and add oil, heat over high heat. Add garlic and chicken and sauté until browned on both sides, season chicken with salt and pepper. Reduce heat to medium low and add chicken broth and lemon juice. Cover skillet and simmer until chicken is cooked through, about 5 to 7 minutes. Remove cover and let simmer another 5 minutes. Serve with sauce spooned over chicken. Garnish with lemon slices and sprinkle with fresh parsley. Great with pasta or rice.

Chicken and Vegetable Stir Fry

10 to 12 chicken tenders
1 teaspoon garlic, minced
2 tablespoons dark sesame oil, divided
2 carrots, sliced
2 stalks celery, sliced
2 cups broccoli florets

1 cup sliced mushrooms
2 green onions, sliced
1 red or yellow pepper, sliced
1 cup chicken broth
2 tablespoons cornstarch
3 cups cooked rice

In a large skillet over medium-high heat, sauté chicken tenders and garlic in 1 tablespoon sesame oil until cooked through. Add other tablespoon sesame oil and vegetables and stir fry until vegetables are semi-tender and bright in color. In a small bowl, whisk chicken broth and cornstarch together. Reduce heat to medium and pour chicken broth mixture over chicken and vegetables and cook until thickened, while stirring constantly. Serve over rice.

Beef Tips over Parsleyed Noodles

1 large yellow onion, chopped
1 cup sliced mushrooms
4 tablespoons margarine
1 cup flour

1 teaspoon salt
3 pounds sirloin tips
2 cups beef broth
salt and pepper to taste

In a large skillet with high sides, melt margarine over medium-high heat. Sauté onions and mushrooms until tender, about 5 minutes. Remove onions and mushrooms from skillet with a slotted spoon, leaving much of the leftover juices and margarine in the skillet.

Mix flour and salt together in a medium-sized bowl. Dredge stew meat in flour mixture until well coated, then sauté in skillet over medium high heat until edges of meat are browned. Add beef broth to meat and simmer over low heat for 20 to 25 minutes until beef is cooked through and tender. Add mushrooms and onion and heat thoroughly. Salt and pepper to taste. Serves 6.

Serve over buttered parsleyed noodles (12 ounces egg noodles, cooked, and while noodles are still hot mix in 2 tablespoons margarine and 1/4 cup parsley).

Potato Cakes with Garlic and Onion

2 pounds red potatoes, washed
    and not peeled
2 teaspoons garlic, chopped
2 green onions, chopped
1 tablespoon fresh parsley,
2 cup chopped
2 tablespoons yellow cornmeal,
    plus extra for coating cakes
    before frying

2 tablespoons margarine
2 tablespoons enriched rice milk
1 egg, or egg substitute, beaten
2 tablespoons olive oil for frying
salt and pepper
all-vegetable cooking spray

Boil potatoes in a large pot of water until tender, rinse, drain, and cool. Return potatoes to pot, add garlic, margarine and rice milk, and mash. Stir in green onion, parsley, and 2 tablespoons cornmeal. Cover and refrigerate until well chilled, 2 to 4 hours.

Form potato mixture into small cakes, dip in beaten egg, coat with cornmeal. Fry in a medium skillet with olive oil over medium-high heat until heated through and golden brown on each side.

May also bake these cakes: preheat oven to 425 degrees, line a baking sheet with foil, brush with olive oil, and place cakes on pan. Bake for 10 minutes on each side, until golden brown and heated through.

Garlic Mashed Potatoes

2 pounds red potatoes, peeled and quartered
2 fourteen-ounce cans chicken broth

2 tablespoons margarine
2 teaspoons garlic, minced
salt and pepper

In a medium saucepan, bring broth to a boil, add potatoes and reduce heat, simmering until potatoes are tender. Drain potatoes, reserving 1/2 cup broth. In a small skillet, melt margarine, then sauté garlic over medium high heat until golden brown. Pour garlic and margarine over potatoes in a large bowl, add chicken broth and mash. Salt and pepper to taste and serve.

Potato and Zucchini Gratin

3 medium potatoes, thinly sliced (russet or Yukon)
1 medium zucchini, thinly sliced
2 teaspoons seasoning salt
2 tablespoons margarine

1/2 cup onion, chopped
1 & 1/2 cups enriched rice milk
2 tablespoons flour
1/4 teaspoon nutmeg
all-vegetable cooking spray

Coat an 8 x 8 inch casserole with cooking spray. Arrange one third of the potatoes over the bottom of the casserole, sprinkle lightly with seasoning salt. Layer one half of the zucchini on top of the potatoes and again sprinkle with seasoning salt. Repeat layering and sprinkling the potatoes and zucchini ending with the potatoes on top. Set aside.

In a medium saucepan, heat the margarine over medium heat to melt. Add the chopped onion and sauté until onion is tender. In a separate small bowl, whisk or blend the rice milk and flour until it is smooth, pour into the saucepan with the onion, and bring to a boil over medium heat while stirring constantly. Remove from heat once sauce just begins to boil. Stir in nutmeg.

Pour the white sauce over the potatoes and zucchini. Cover with foil and bake for 40 minutes at 350 degrees. Uncover and bake 10 to 15 minutes more, until golden brown.

Spinach and Rice Gratin

1 cup dry white rice
1 1/2 cups chicken broth
1 ten-ounce package frozen
    chopped spinach, thawed
    and squeezed dry
2 tablespoons margarine
1/2 cup onion, chopped
1/2 teaspoon minced garlic

1 cup mushrooms, sliced
1 cup enriched rice milk
2 tablespoons flour
1/2 cup egg substitute
1 teaspoon salt
1/2 teaspoon pepper
all-vegetable cooking spray

In a medium saucepan, bring chicken broth to a boil. Add rice, reduce to simmer, and cover until rice is tender, about 35 minutes.

In a medium skillet, melt margarine, then sauté onion and garlic until onion is tender, about 5 minutes. Add mushrooms and continue to sauté for 5 minutes. In a large bowl, mix together spinach and onion/mushroom mixture. Mix in rice. In a separate small bowl, whisk together rice milk, flour and egg substitute. Pour over rice mixture and stir to blend.

Pour into a 13 x 9-inch casserole coated with cooking spray. Bake, uncovered, at 350 degrees until set, and light golden brown, 35-45 minutes.

Red Beans and Rice

4 cups cooked white rice
2 tablespoons olive oil
1 medium onion, chopped
1 teaspoon garlic, minced

3 fifteen-ounce cans kidney
beans, undrained
1 & 1/2 cups chicken broth
1-2 teaspoons Cajun seasoning,
to taste

Heat oil in a large skillet with high sides. Sauté onion and garlic over medium-high heat until onion is tender and golden brown. Pour in kidney beans, chicken broth, and seasoning. Cover and simmer over reduced heat for 50 minutes to an hour. Spoon over rice and serve. Serves 4-6.

Lemon Bars

Crust:
1/2 cup sugar
6 tablespoons margarine, softened
1 & 3/4 cups all-purpose flour
Filling:
5 eggs

1 & 1/2 cups sugar
1 tablespoon grated lemon rind
1/2 cup fresh lemon juice
5 tablespoons all-purpose flour
1 teaspoon baking powder
1/4 teaspoon salt
powdered sugar for garnish

Preheat oven to 350 degrees. Mix first three ingredients together until mixture is crumbly (a food processor works well for this). Press mixture into the bottom of a 13 x 9-inch pan and bake for 15 to 18 minutes. Cool. Beat eggs with an electric mixer until foamy and lemon colored. Add sugar and beat well. Then add lemon rind, lemon juice, flour, baking powder and salt. Beat until well blended. Pour lemon mixture over crust and bake at 350 degrees for 20 to 25 minutes, until set. Cool, then sprinkle powdered sugar. Makes 20-24 bars.

Gravy and Sauces

Chicken Gravy

2 tablespoons margarine
2 cups chicken broth
1/2 teaspoon cinnamon
1/8 teaspoon nutmeg

3 tablespoons flour
salt and pepper
1/2 teaspoon cinnamon
1 tablespoon margarine

Melt margarine in a medium saucepan. Add 1 cup chicken broth to 2 tablespoons flour and blend until smooth (or may be shaken to mix in an airtight container). Into the saucepan over medium heat, add remaining 1 cup chicken broth and flour/chicken broth mixture. Stir constantly while mixture heats and just begins to boil. Remove from heat. Season to taste with salt and pepper. Serve.

*This recipe can made substituting vegetable, beef, fish stock, or turkey broth as well.

Clear Chicken Gravy, or Glaze

2 tablespoons margarine
2 cups chicken broth

1 tablespoon cornstarch
dash salt

Melt the margarine in a medium saucepan. Combine 1 cup chicken broth with cornstarch and blend until smooth. Pour remaining cup chicken broth and cornstarch mixture into the saucepan. Over medium heat, cook until mixture just begins to boil, while stirring constantly. Remove from heat. Season with salt to taste.

Mushroom Gravy

1/2 pound fresh mushrooms,
   sliced
2 tablespoons margarine

1/2 teaspoon minced garlic
2 cups beef broth
2 tablespoons cornstarch

    Over medium heat in a non-stick skillet, sauté the mushrooms and garlic in margarine. Combine the beef broth and cornstarch in a small bowl and blend, or whisk until smooth. Pour the beef broth and cornstarch mixture into a medium saucepan placed over medium heat and stir until the mixture begins to boil. Remove from heat and add mushrooms and garlic. Season with salt and pepper to taste.

Basic White Sauce (Bechamel)

2 tablespoons margarine
2 cups enriched rice milk

3 tablespoons flour
salt and pepper

    Melt margarine in a medium saucepan. Combine rice milk and flour and blend until smooth. Pour rice milk/flour mixture into saucepan and increase heat to medium. Stir constantly until mixture just begins to boil. Remove from heat. Salt and pepper to taste.

    **Rice milk is very thin, and lacks the body that 2 percent or whole milk has; therefore it does not stand up to high temperatures well. When making sauces with thickener, allow mixture to boil only briefly and then remove from heat. The sauce will keep a thicker consistency.

Lemon Dill Sauce

1 recipe basic white sauce
1/8 cup fresh dill, chopped

juice of 1/2 lemon

    Prepare basic white sauce and whisk in lemon and dill. Season with salt to taste. This sauce is good over fish.

Pesto

Pesto is great over pasta, or spread lightly on bread and grilled. Most pesto recipes contain parmesan cheese; these are lighter and milk-free.

Basil Pesto

1 cup fresh basil leaves
3 garlic cloves, peeled
1/4 cup pine nuts

1/4 cup fresh lemon juice
1/8 cup olive oil

Place all ingredients in a food processor or blender. Process until mixture becomes a smooth paste. Makes 1/2 cup. Use 1/4 cup over 8 ounces of pasta. Pesto freezes well.

Cilantro Pesto

1 cup fresh cilantro
3 garlic cloves, peeled
1/4 cup walnuts

1/8 cup fresh lemon juice
1/8 cup olive oil

Place all ingredients in a food processor or blender. Process until mixture becomes a smooth paste. Makes 1/2 cup.

Meatless Dishes

Black Bean Burgers

3 fifteen-ounce cans black beans,
   undrained
3 cups cooked brown rice
1 medium onion, diced
2 teaspoons chopped garlic
1 tablespoon olive oil

1 teaspoon chile powder
1 teaspoon salt
1 & 1/2 cups bread crumbs
3 tablespoons minced cilantro
Olive oil or all-vegetable cooking
   spray for frying

Heat oil in large skillet on medium-high heat. Add garlic and onion and sauté until onion is softened, about 5 minutes. In a large food processor, process rice and beans until blended, but not puréed, about 1 minute. Place bean mixture into a large bowl. Add onion, garlic, chile powder and salt and stir until blended. Stir in bread crumbs and cilantro.

Shape bean mixture into patties and fry in a small amount of olive oil or cooking spray.

Serve burgers as you would hamburgers. These burgers freeze well if you wrap them individually and then store them in an airtight container. Makes 12 large burgers.

BBQ Baked Bean Burgers

3 fifteen-ounce cans vegetarian
   baked beans, undrained
3 cups cooked brown rice
1 medium onion, chopped
2 teaspoons chopped garlic
2 tablespoons olive oil

2 tablespoons barbeque sauce
   (your favorite)
1 teaspoon salt
3 cups bread crumbs
Olive oil or cooking spray for
   frying

Heat oil in a medium skillet over medium-high heat. Sauté onion and garlic until onion is softened, about 5 minutes.

In a large food processor, process rice and beans until blended, but not smooth. Add onion and garlic, salt, and barbeque sauce until just blended. Place bean mixture in a large mixing bowl. Add bread crumbs to bean mixture and blend.

Shape bean mixture into patties and fry until golden brown. Serve as you would hamburgers. Makes 12 large burgers.

Brown Rice Burgers

2 cups mushrooms, sliced
1 cup celery, chopped
1 & 1/2 cups carrots, chopped
1 large onion, chopped
2 tablespoons garlic, chopped
1/2 stick margarine
2 cubes chicken bouillon

1/3 cup boiling water
2 teaspoons Lawry's seasoning salt
4 cups cooked brown rice
2 eggs
1/2 cup Malt O'Meal® cereal, uncooked

Heat olive oil in a large skillet over medium-high heat. Add garlic and onion, and sauté until just browned. Add mushrooms, celery and carrots, and sauté until softened. Cool mixture. When cooled, purée mixture in food processor until mixture appears grated, but still some chunks remain. Set aside. In a large bowl, mix rice with 2 beaten eggs. In a separate small bowl, mix boiling water and bouillon cubes and stir until dissolved. Add bouillon mixture and seasoning salt to the rice mixture and stir to blend, then add vegetable mixture and mix well. Let stand for 15 minutes.

Heat a large non-stick skillet to medium heat. Form the rice mixture into burger-sized patties and brown on each side. Serve with hamburger buns, lettuce, tomato, pickle, onion and other condiments. Makes 18-20 burgers.

Roasted Vegetable Burgers

3 cups water
2 chicken or vegetable bouillon
    cubes
3/4 cup brown rice
1/2 cup brown lentils, rinsed and
    drained
1/3 cup cracked wheat
1/2 cup roasted red peppers,
    chopped

1/2 cup green onion, chopped
1 cup mushrooms, chopped
1 teaspoon garlic, minced
1 tablespoon olive oil
1 teaspoon oregano
2 eggs
1/2 cup flour
salt and pepper
all-vegetable cooking spray

Bring the water to a boil in a medium saucepan. Add bouillon, rice, lentils, and cracked wheat. Stir to dissolve and mix in bouillon, cover, and reduce to low heat. Cook 40 to 45 minutes until tender, or moisture is evaporated. Remove from heat and cool.

In a heavy skillet, heat olive oil over medium-high heat. Add garlic, and sauté 1 to 2 minutes until light golden brown. Add mushrooms, peppers and green onions, and sauté 5 to 6 minutes. Remove from heat, stir on oregano, and cool.

When above mixtures are cool, stir them together in a large bowl. Season to taste with salt and pepper. Mix in eggs and flour. Form mixture into patties and turn into a heavy skillet coated with all-vegetable cooking spray. Lightly fry patties for 3 to 4 minutes on each side until they are golden brown. Serve as you would hamburgers.

Pinto Bean and Potato Burritos

10 large (10-inch round) flour
    tortillas
2 fifteen and a half ounce cans
    vegetarian refried pinto
    beans
3 medium baking potatoes

2 medium green onions
1 four-ounce can diced green
    chiles
seasoning salt or salt-free season-
    ing
all-vegetable cooking spray
salsa

Pierce the potatoes several times with a fork, then microwave for 10 minutes on high, stopping at five minutes to turn potatoes one-quarter turn. Set the potatoes aside and allow to cool. In a medium-sized saucepan, heat the refried beans and green chiles over low heat. When the potatoes are cool enough to handle, dice them into 1/2-inch pieces.

Place a large skillet over medium-high heat, spray with cooking spray, then add potatoes and green onion. Sauté the potato mixture until the potatoes are golden brown. Season, and remove from heat.

Fold the potato mixture into the refried beans and stir to blend. Fill each of the flour tortillas with 1/2 cup of the bean mixture, add salsa, and serve. May be garnished with fresh tomato, black olives, shredded lettuce, guacamole and cilantro.

Black Bean Enchilada Bake

1 cup cooked brown rice
1 fifteen-ounce can black beans, drained
1 cup egg substitute
1/2 cup green onions, chopped
1/4 cup fresh cilantro, chopped
1 four-ounce can diced green chiles
1 four-ounce can sliced black olives, drained
1/2 teaspoon salt
1 nineteen-ounce can red enchilada sauce (you may want to use the powdered mix; some canned sauce contains soy protein).
4 cups bite-sized tortilla chips

In a large bowl, mix together the first ten ingredients. Spray a 13 x 9-inch casserole dish with all-vegetable cooking spray. Place 2 cups tortilla chips on the bottom of the casserole, then top with half the bean and rice mixture. Repeat layering again. Bake at 350 degrees for 40 to 45 minutes.

This casserole is best served for the first time. Make a little extra sauce for leftovers; it tends to get dryer with each reheating.

Side Dishes

Creamed Mushrooms and Artichokes

2 fourteen-ounce cans quartered
    artichoke hearts, drained
1 pound fresh mushrooms,
    washed and halved
1 cup enriched rice milk

2 teaspoons instant chicken
    bouillon granules
2 tablespoons margarine
1/4 cup green onions, chopped
2 tablespoons flour
dash nutmeg
1/2 cup pecans, chopped

In a microwave-safe dish, combine artichokes and mushrooms, cover with plastic wrap, and cook in a microwave set on high for 8 to 10 minutes. Drain.

In a medium saucepan over medium heat, melt margarine. Sauté green onions for 1 to 2 minutes. In a small bowl, whisk flour and bouillon granules into rice milk. Pour rice milk mixture into saucepan and cook over medium high heat while stirring constantly. Remove mixture from heat when thickened and just beginning to boil. Stir in nutmeg.

Pour white sauce over mushrooms and artichokes in medium microwave-safe dish. Place in microwave oven and heat for 2 to 3 minutes on high, stopping to stir every minute. Top with pecans and serve.

Sautéed Zucchini and Summer Squash with Chile and Lime

1 medium zucchini, rinsed and
    sliced
1 medium yellow crooknecked
    squash, rinsed and sliced

1/2 teaspoon chile powder
1 lime
1/4 teaspoon salt
all-vegetable cooking spray

Heat a medium skillet to medium-high heat, and coat with cooking spray. Add zucchini and squash and sauté until tender, about 5 minutes. Remove from heat, squeeze the juice of one lime over top, and stir. Sprinkle with chile powder and salt and serve. This recipe works well with grilled zucchini too.

Glazed Carrots

1 pound whole baby carrots
2 tablespoons margarine
1/4 cup orange juice concentrate

1/2 cup packed brown sugar
salt and pepper to taste
dash nutmeg

Place carrots in a large saucepan and cover with water. Bring to a boil and simmer until carrots are tender, about 25 to 30 minutes. Drain carrots in a colander. In a separate small saucepan, heat margarine until melted, adding brown sugar and orange juice concentrate. Once mixture is melted, heat thoroughly over medium heat until sugar is completely dissolved. Pour sauce over carrots, salt and pepper to taste, and add a dash of nutmeg.

Breads and Muffins

Honey Oatmeal Bread

4 cups water	3 packages yeast
2 1/2 cups oatmeal	1/2 cup warm water
2 sticks margarine	1 teaspoon salt
1 cup honey, plus 1 teaspoonful for yeast	7 cups flour, plus extra flour for kneading
3 cups all-purpose flour	all-vegetable cooking spray

Bring 4 cups water to a boil, add oatmeal and simmer until fully cooked. Cool slightly and add margarine and honey. Mix in 3 cups flour.

Whisk the yeast and 1 tablespoon honey into 1/2 cup warm (not hot) water. Let mixture foam up slightly to proof, then mix into oatmeal batter. Mix in remaining flour, 1 cup at a time, using a heavy duty mixer or a large food processor. You may have to knead in the remaining 1 to 2 cups flour. The dough will be a little soft; you may add a bit more flour to make it easier to handle, but not so much that the dough becomes stiff.

Let the dough rise in a large bowl coated with cooking spray, covering the top of the bowl with a light cloth. Let rise until doubled in size. When dough has doubled, punch it down and divide into 4 separate loaves. Place dough in loaf pans coated with cooking spray, cover and again let rise. Bake in an oven preheated to 350 degrees for 40 to 50 minutes. Let the loaves cool on wire racks. When completely cool, remove bread from pans.

Option: Cinnamon Rolls

Once the dough has risen for the first time, punch down and separate the dough into 2 equal pieces. Roll each out on a floured work surface into the shape of a large rectangle. Spread 1/2 stick of softened margarine over each rectangle with fingertips. In a small bowl, mix 1 cup brown sugar and 1 tablespoon cinnamon; divide in equal portions and sprinkle over margarine.

Roll the dough lengthwise, taking care to fold in all the toppings, then crimp the edges so it will stay in place. Slice the rolls in 1 & 1/2-inch portions. Place the rolls into glass baking dishes coated with cooking spray. Cover and let rise until doubled in size. Bake the rolls in a 325-degree oven for 20 to 25 minutes, until they are light golden brown. Cool, then frost (frosting recipe on page 74).

Pumpkin Bread (*makes 2 loaves*)

1 stick margarine, softened
1 & 1/2 cups sugar
1/2 cup brown sugar
4 eggs, or egg substitute
1 fifteen-ounce can pumpkin pu-
    ree ·
1 teaspoon vanilla
2/3 cup enriched rice milk
1/4 cup canola oil

3 & 1/2 cups all-purpose flour
2 teaspoons baking soda
1 teaspoon baking powder
1/2 teaspoon salt
1 teaspoon ground cinnamon
1/2 teaspoon ground ginger
1/4 teaspoon ground nutmeg
1/4 teaspoon ground cloves

Preheat the oven to 350 degrees. Cream together margarine and sugars. Add eggs, one at a time, beating after each addition. Mix in vanilla, pumpkin, rice milk, and canola oil. Stir in flour, baking soda, powder and spices. Pour batter into loaf pans coated with cooking spray. Bake 50 to 60 minutes, until a tester comes out clean. Cool 10 minutes, run a knife around edge of pans and then remove loaves.

Banana Bread

1 stick margarine, softened
1 cup sugar
2 eggs
2 cups all-purpose flour
1 teaspoon baking soda

1/2 teaspoon salt
3 ripe bananas, mashed
1 teaspoon vanilla
all-vegetable cooking spray

Preheat oven to 350 degrees. Cream margarine and sugar together. Add eggs and beat 1 to 2 minutes. Mix in flour, baking soda and salt. Stir in mashed banana and vanilla. Pour batter into a 9 x 5-inch loaf pan coated with cooking spray. Bake for 45 to 55 minutes, until a toothpick inserted in the center comes out clean. Cool loaf pan for 10 minutes, then remove and cool on wire rack.

Apple Bread

1 stick margarine, softened
1 cup sugar
1/2 cup packed brown sugar
2 eggs
1 teaspoon vanilla

1 & 1/2 cups shredded apples,
    such as Granny Smith
juice of 1/2 lemon
2 cups all-purpose flour
1/2 teaspoon baking soda
1/2 teaspoon cinnamon
all-vegetable cooking spray

Cream margarine and sugars together. Add eggs and beat until smooth. Stir in vanilla. Grate apple and toss with lemon juice, set aside. Mix all the dry ingredients together and stir into batter. Add apples and stir until moistened. Pour batter into a 9 x 5-inch loaf pan coated with cooking spray. Bake at 350 degrees for 50 to 60 minutes, or until a tester comes out clean. Cool for 10 minutes, then turn out to cool on a wire rack.

Chocolate Marble Bread

1 & 1/4 cups sugar
1 & 1/2 sticks margarine, soft-
    ened
1 & 1/2 cups all-purpose flour
1/2 cup enriched rice milk
1/2 teaspoon baking powder

1/4 teaspoon baking soda
1/2 teaspoon salt
2 large eggs
1/4 cup cocoa powder
all-vegetable cooking spray

Coat a 9 x 5-inch loaf pan with cooking spray and set aside. Preheat oven to 350 degrees. In a large bowl, beat together margarine and sugar until light and fluffy. Reduce speed to low and mix in flour, rice milk, baking powder, baking soda and salt. Beat in eggs one at a time.

Remove 1/2 of the batter and place in a smaller bowl. Beat the cocoa into the batter remaining in larger bowl. Alternately spoon the chocolate and vanilla batters into the loaf pan, then, using a knife, cut through the batters to marble.

Bake for 50 to 60 minutes, or until a tester comes out clean. Cool 10 minutes in loaf pan, then remove to cool on wire rack.

Orange Cranberry Nut Bread

1 stick margarine, softened
1 cup sugar
1 egg
3/4 cup enriched rice milk
1/2 cup orange juice
1 tablespoon grated orange peel
2 cups all-purpose flour

1/2 teaspoon baking soda
1/2 teaspoon baking powder
1 teaspoon salt
1/2 cup chopped pecans
1 & 1/2 cups dried cranberries
all-vegetable cooking spray

Preheat oven to 350 degrees. Cream margarine and sugar together. Add egg and beat in until smooth. Stir in orange juice and orange peel. Mix flour, baking soda and powder and salt together. Mix dry ingredients in alternately with rice milk. Stir in pecans and cranberries. Pour batter into a 9 x 5-inch loaf pan coated with cooking spray. Bake for 50 to 60 minutes, or until a tester comes out clean. Cool for 10 minutes, then remove from pan.

Lemon Bread (*makes 2 loaves*)

1 stick margarine
1 & 1/2 cups sugar
2 large eggs and 1 egg white
1/4 cup canola oil
1/2 cup enriched rice milk
1/2 cup lemon juice

2 tablespoons grated lemon rind
2 cups all-purpose flour
1 & 1/2 teaspoons baking powder
1/4 teaspoon salt
all-vegetable cooking spray

Cream the margarine and sugar together until fluffy. Beat in eggs and egg white, oil and lemon rind. Mix in dry ingredients alternately with lemon juice and rice milk. Pour batter into 2 loaf pans coated with cooking spray. Bake at 350 degrees for 35 to 45 minutes, or until a tester come out clean. Cool 10 minutes; loosen edges with a knife before removing from pan.

Bran Muffins

2 & 1/2 cups all-purpose flour
1 & 3/4 cups sugar
2 teaspoons baking powder
1/2 teaspoon baking soda
1/2 teaspoon salt
2 cups enriched rice milk
1/4 cup canola oil

1 #2 jar baby food prunes, or 1/2
 cup of your favorite jam
2 eggs
8 cups bran flakes
optional: 1/2 cup chopped nuts,
 cinnamon raisins, or other
 dried fruit

Preheat the oven to 350 degrees. Line muffin cups with paper liners. Whisk rice milk, oil, prunes, and eggs together. Add dry ingredients and cereal until well-blended. Add other optional ingredients at this time as well. Spoon mixture into muffin cups until 3/4ths full. Bake for 25 minutes, or until a tester comes out clean. Place muffins on wire racks to cool.

Banana Nut Muffins

2 ripe bananas, mashed
1 stick margarine, melted
1 egg
2 & 1/2 tablespoons enriched vanilla rice milk

1 & 1/2 cups all-purpose flour
3/4 cup sugar
1 & 1/2 teaspoons baking soda
1/4 teaspoon salt
1/2 cup chopped nuts

Preheat the oven to 350 degrees. Line muffin cups with paper liners. Mix dry ingredients together and set aside. Combine bananas, margarine, rice milk, and egg, whisking to blend. Add banana mixture to dry ingredients and blend well. Spoon batter into muffin cups, filling only 3/4ths full. Bake for 25 minutes, or until a tester comes out clean. Cool on wire rack.

Brunch Dishes

Florentine Eggs

1 package frozen chopped spinach, thawed and squeezed of
  excess moisture
10 eggs, or egg substitute
1/4 cup melted margarine

1 cup turkey, or regular pepperoni, diced
1 & 1/2 cups enriched rice milk
4 cups cubed bread, with crusts
  removed
1/2 teaspoon salt

Preheat the oven to 350 degrees. Whisk eggs and rice milk in a large
mixing bowl. Add spinach and pepperoni and stir. Add bread cubes and
mix well. Pour egg mixture into a 13 x 9-inch casserole coated with cooking spray. (This casserole may be baked immediately or refrigerated for
several hours before baking).
  Bake for 45 to 50 minutes, until puffed and golden brown.

Vegetable Strata

2 tablespoons olive oil
2 cups mushrooms, sliced
2 cups zucchini, chopped
1 cup orange bell pepper,
  chopped
1 cup sweet onion, such as
  Vidalia, chopped
2 teaspoons garlic, chopped

1 fourteen-ounce can artichoke
  hearts, drained and chopped
1 cup Roma tomatoes, chopped
8 cups French bread, crusts
  trimmed and cubed
8 eggs, or egg substitute
1 & 1/2 cups enriched rice milk
2 teaspoons seasoning salt, such
  as Lawrys
1/2 teaspoon dry mustard
all-vegetable cooking spray

In a large skillet, sauté mushrooms, zucchini, bell pepper, onion and
garlic in olive oil. Sauté for 6 to 8 minutes until vegetables are tender. Set
aside to cool. When cool, add artichokes and tomatoes.

Coat a 13 x 9-inch baking dish with cooking spray. Preheat oven to 350 degrees. Place cubed bread in the baking dish. In a medium bowl, whisk together eggs, rice milk, salt and dry mustard.

Pour cooled vegetables over the top of the bread, then pour egg mixture over top. Cover and refrigerate for a couple of hours, or overnight. Bake for 50 to 60 minutes, or until bubbly and golden brown.

Zucchini-Potato Frittata

8 eggs
2 tablespoons enriched rice milk
2 tablespoons margarine
1 medium zucchini, diced

1 medium red potato, diced
2 teaspoons Italian seasoning
all-vegetable cooking spray

Preheat oven to broil. In a medium bowl, beat eggs with rice milk. Set aside. Heat a 10-inch non-stick skillet to medium-high heat. Add margarine and melt. Sauté zucchini and potato until lightly browned. Sprinkle on seasoning. Reduce heat to medium and add egg mixture. As eggs begin to cook, lift the edges with a spatula so the uncooked eggs will flow underneath and cook. Repeat until the egg mixture is cooked. Transfer to a pie plate, coated with cooking spray. Broil 3 to 4 minutes until top is golden brown. Remove, cool, and serve.

Southwest Strata

1 cup enriched rice milk
4 eggs
1 green onion, chopped
2 tablespoons diced green chiles

2 cups white bread, torn into
bite-sized pieces
all-vegetable cooking spray

Preheat oven to 400 degrees. Coat a 10-inch quiche or pie plate with cooking spray. Whisk together rice milk and eggs. Stir in green onion and green chiles. Add bread and stir until well blended. Transfer mixture into prepared baking dish. Let egg mixture set so bread can soak up moisture, about 10 minutes.

Bake, uncovered, until lightly browned, and puffed up, about 25 to 30 minutes. Serve with salsa.

Overnight French Toast

1 cup packed brown sugar
1 stick margarine
1 tablespoon light corn syrup
12 slices white bread, crusts re-
    moved (about 12 oz. bread)

1 & 1/2 cups enriched vanilla
    rice milk
6 large eggs (egg substitute may
    be used)
1/4 teaspoon salt
2 teaspoons cinnamon
all-vegetable cooking spray

Combine brown sugar, margarine and corn syrup in small saucepan. Bring to a boil over medium heat while stirring constantly. Allow mixture to boil 5 minutes still slightly thickened. Pour mixture into a 13 x 9-inch pan, coated with cooking spray, and spread until mixture covers the bottom of the pan.

Arrange bread slices over the brown sugar mixture in pan, double layering bread. Whisk eggs, rice milk, cinnamon and salt. Pour over bread. Cover and refrigerate overnight. Bake at 350 degrees until light golden brown and bread is puffed. Let cool 10 minutes, then serve warm. Invert servings onto dessert plates so the caramel sauce runs over the bread. Great with Cranberry Salsa.

**Variations: add 1/2 cup chopped pecans, raisins, or dried cranberries to the caramel layer before adding bread.

Cranberry Salsa

1 can crushed pineapple, drained
2 cans mandarin oranges, drained

1 can whole cranberry sauce
1/2 cup chopped walnuts

Mix fruit and nuts together. Chill before serving.

Pancakes

1 cup all-purpose flour
1 teaspoon baking soda
1/4 teaspoon salt
1 & 1/4 teaspoon salt

1 & 1/4 cups rice milk
2 tablespoons margarine, melted
1 egg

Combine dry ingredients in a medium mixing bowl. In a small bowl, whisk together rice milk, margarine, and egg. Add to flour mixture and stir until smooth. Heat a non-stick griddle over medium-high heat. Spoon batter onto griddle. Turn when tops of pancakes are all bubbly. Makes 10 to 12 pancakes. Serve with margarine and syrup.

**Variations: use enriched vanilla rice milk instead of original flavor, add 1 teaspoon cinnamon.

Cinnamon French Toast

2 eggs
3/4 cup enriched vanilla rice milk
1 teaspoon cinnamon

1/4 teaspoon nutmeg
8 slices thick French bread
confectioners' sugar

Whisk together eggs, rice milk, and spices. Heat a non-stick skillet over medium-high heat. Dip bread slices in egg mixture, then place in skillet. Cook until golden brown on each side, turning once. Arrange on plate, dust with confectioners' powder.

**Great served with sliced bananas and maple syrup.

Desserts: Cookies, Cakes, and Comfort Foods

Monster Cookies

1 & 1/2 cups brown sugar
1 stick margarine
1 cup peanut butter
3 eggs
1 & 1/2 cups flour
1 cup sugar

2 teaspoons baking soda
1/2 teaspoon salt
2 teaspoons vanilla
4 cups rolled oats
6 ounces semi-sweet chocolate
   chips, or chocolate chunks

Cream first 3 ingredients together, then add eggs one at a time, beating after each addition. Mix in sugar, flour, baking soda, salt and vanilla. Stir in rolled oats, then chocolate. Spoon dough onto cookie sheets in heaping tablespoons. Bake at 350 degrees for 10-12 minutes. Cookies should be light brown. Remove pan from oven and let cookies sit on pan for an additional 2 minutes before removing.

**May add chopped nuts, raisins or cinnamon raisins, as you wish. These cookies freeze well in an airtight container for at least one month. Freezing them the same day as you bake them keeps them very fresh and chewy. They thaw quickly when removed one at a time for snacking! These are my most favorite cookie!

Chocolate Chocolate-Chip Walnut Cookies

1/2 stick margarine
2/3 cup packed brown sugar
2 eggs
2/3 cup all-purpose flour
1/4 teaspoon baking powder
1 teaspoon vanilla

1/4 teaspoon salt
1 twelve-ounce package
   semi-sweet chocolate chips,
   divided
1 cup chopped walnuts

Preheat oven to 350 degrees. Place 6 ounces chocolate chips in a microwave-safe bowl and cook on high for 1 to 2 minutes, until chocolate is melted, stopping to stir every 30 seconds. Mix melted chocolate together with margarine, brown sugar, eggs and vanilla. Mix in flour, baking powder and salt. Stir in remaining chocolate chips and walnuts.

Drop cookies onto a cookie sheet by teaspoonfuls. Bake 11 to 12 minutes or until puffed and set. Cool on cookie sheet for 2 minutes then remove and cool.

Cranberry Orange Oatmeal Cookies

2 sticks margarine, softened
1 cup sugar
1 cup packed brown sugar
2 eggs
1 teaspoon vanilla
1 tablespoon orange zest, grated

2 cups all-purpose flour
1 teaspoon baking soda
1/2 teaspoon salt
3 cups rolled oats
*2 cups (12 ounces) dried cranberries

Preheat oven to 350 degrees. Mix together margarine and sugars until smooth, then add eggs, and blend thoroughly. Mix in vanilla and orange zest. In a separate bowl, mix flour, baking soda and salt together. Add flour mixture to the dough and stir until well blended. Stir in oats and cranberries. Drop by teaspoonfuls onto cookie sheets and bake 10-12 minutes until light golden brown. Leave cookies to cool on pan for 2 minutes then remove to a wire rack. Makes 4-5 dozen.

*You may substitute diced dates or prunes (I love the orange scented prunes in these cookies), or other diced dried fruit. Raisins, cinnamon raisins or chocolate chips are also great. (when adding chocolate chips, you may take out the orange zest, or leave it in for a great flavor treat!)

Oatmeal Chip Cookies

2 sticks margarine, softened
1 cup sugar
1 cup packed brown sugar
1 egg
2 teaspoons vanilla
2 cups all-purpose flour
1 teaspoon baking soda

1/2 teaspoon salt
1 teaspoon cinnamon
1/4 teaspoon nutmeg
3 cups rolled oats
1 twelve-ounce package chocolate chips

Preheat oven to 375 degrees. Cream margarine and sugars until creamy and smooth. Mix in egg and vanilla. Add flour, salt, soda and spices and mix thoroughly. Stir in oats and chocolate chips. Drop by rounded teaspoons onto cookie sheets and bake 9-10 minutes. Cool 2 minutes on cookie sheets. Makes 4-5 dozen cookies. Store in airtight container or freeze after cooling for longer freshness.

Ginger Cream Cookies

1 & 1/2 sticks margarine, softened
2 cups sugar, plus extra sugar for
   rolling cookies
1/2 cup molasses
2 eggs
2 teaspoons vanilla extract

4 cups all-purpose flour
4 teaspoons baking soda
1 teaspoon salt
1 teaspoon ground ginger
2 teaspoons ground cinnamon
1/4 teaspoon ground nutmeg
1 teaspoon ground cloves

Preheat oven to 350 degrees. Cream together margarine and sugar. Mix in molasses, eggs and vanilla until well blended. Mix in flour, baking soda, salt, and spices. Roll dough into 1-inch balls and roll in sugar. Bake for 8 to 10 minutes, until cookies are flat and have a cracked appearance. Cool and frost. Makes about 5 dozen cookies.

Frosting:

2 tablespoons margarine, soft-
    ened

2 cups powdered sugar
1 teaspoon vanilla
2-3 tablespoons enriched rice
    milk
red food coloring

Combine first 3 ingredients and mix until smooth. Add 2 tablespoons rice milk and mix well; if frosting is too stiff, add more rice milk. Add a drop or two of red food coloring if desired, so the frosting becomes light pink in color.

Snickerdoodles

2 sticks margarine, softened
1 & 1/2 cups sugar
2 eggs
3 & 1/4 cups flour
2 teaspoons cream of tartar

1 teaspoon baking soda
1/2 teaspoon salt
1/2 cup sugar and 3 tablespoons
    cinnamon for garnish

Cream margarine and sugar together. Add eggs, one at a time, and beat after each addition. Mix dry ingredients (flour, cream of tartar, baking soda and salt) into batter. Chill dough about an hour. In a small bowl mix together sugar and cinnamon. Roll dough into small (1-inch) balls and roll in sugar and cinnamon. Bake until very lightly browned, about 10 to 12 minutes in an oven preheated to 400 degrees. Cookies will puff up slightly and then flatten down.

Pecan Snowballs

2 sticks margarine, softened
1/2 cup sugar
2 teaspoons vanilla
1 teaspoon salt

2 cups all-purpose flour
1 cup finely chopped pecans
powdered sugar for garnish

Cream margarine and sugar together. Mix in vanilla, then mix in salt and flour. Once dough is well blended, mix in pecans. Roll into small

(1-inch) balls and bake in a 325-degree oven for 20 minutes. When first removed from the oven and cool enough to handle, roll in powdered sugar. After cookies have cooled for 15 to 20 minutes, roll again in powdered sugar.

Peanut Blossom Cookies

1 stick margarine, softened
1/2 cup sugar
1/2 cup brown sugar, packed
1/2 cup peanut butter
1 egg
1 teaspoon vanilla

1 teaspoon baking soda
1 teaspoon salt
2 & 1/4 cups all-purpose flour
sugar for garnish
large semi-sweet chocolate chips
    for garnish, optional

Cream together margarine, sugars, and peanut butter. Add eggs, beating well. Mix in vanilla, flour, baking soda and salt. Roll dough into 1-inch balls (may need to chill dough first), then roll in sugar. Bake in an oven heated to 375 degrees for 10 minutes. Remove cookies from oven and decorate immediately with chocolate chips. Cool on pan 2 minutes, then remove.

Macaroons

1 fourteen-ounce package flaked
    coconut
3/4 cup sugar
1/2 cup all purpose flour

1/2 teaspoon salt
4 large egg whites
1 teaspoon almond extract
1 teaspoon vanilla extract

Mix coconut, sugar, flour, and salt in a medium mixing bowl. In a separate bowl, lightly beat egg whites, and then stir into coconut mixture. Blend well. Mix in almond and vanilla extracts. Drop by rounded teaspoonfuls onto cookie sheets. In an oven preheated to 325 degrees, bake for 20 minutes or until cookies are light golden brown. Remove from cookie sheets and cool on wire racks. Makes approximately 2 dozen.

Option: Mix in 1 cup of semi-sweet chocolate chips before baking.

Almond Meringue Cookies

2 large egg whites   1 teaspoon vanilla
1 cup sugar   1/2 teaspoon almond flavoring
1 cup all-purpose flour   1 cup slivered almonds

Beat egg whites until stiff, then add sugar and continue beating until it is well incorporated. Fold in flour. Stir in vanilla and almond flavorings and slivered almonds. Drop in rounded teaspoons onto cookie sheet lined with waxed paper. Bake in an oven preheated to 350 degrees for 10 to 12 minutes. Cool completely, then carefully remove cookies from waxed paper.

Chocolate Meringues

3 large egg whites   2 tablespoons flour
1 cup sugar   1 teaspoon vanilla extract
4 tablespoons cocoa powder

Beat egg whites until frothy, add sugar slowly until all sugar is beaten in and mixture is stiff. Fold in cocoa, flour and vanilla. Line cookie sheets with waxed paper. Preheat oven to 325 degrees. Drop in rounded teaspoons onto cookie sheets, or you may use a piping or decorating bag fitted with a star tip, and press out 1-inch stars. Bake for 14 to 16 minutes, let cool completely, then carefully remove cookies from waxed paper.

Mocha Meringues

3 large egg whites   1/2 teaspoon instant coffee gran-
1 cup sugar   ules
3 & 1/2 tablespoons cocoa powder   2 tablespoons flour
                                            1 teaspoon vanilla extract

Beat egg whites until frothy, then add sugar gradually until incorporated and mixture is stiff. Fold in cocoa, coffee granules, flour and vanilla. Drop by teaspoons onto cookie sheets lined with waxed paper and bake in an oven preheated to 325 degrees for 14 to 16 minutes. Cool completely, then carefully remove cookies from waxed paper.

Brownies

4 ounces semi-sweet chocolate
    chips, or chopped
    semi-sweet chocolate bars
1 & 1/2 sticks margarine
1 & 1/2 cups sugar
1/2 cup brown sugar

3 eggs, beaten
1 teaspoon vanilla
1 cup all-purpose flour
1/2 cup walnuts, optional
all-vegetable cooking spray

Preheat oven to 350 degrees. In small microwave-safe bowl, melt chocolate chips and margarine on high for 1 minute. Remove from microwave and stir; if chocolate chips are not all melted, return to microwave for another 30 seconds, remove and stir. Place sugars in a large mixing bowl and pour chocolate mixture over top. Mix or stir until sugar is well incorporated. Beat in eggs. Mix in vanilla, flour, and nuts. Pour into 13 x 9-inch baking pan coated with cooking spray. Bake for 30 to 35 minutes until a toothpick comes out clean. Makes 20 to 24 brownies.

Peanut Butter Brownies

1 stick margarine, softened
1 cup creamy peanut butter
1 cup brown sugar
1/2 cup sugar
2 eggs
1/3 cup enriched vanilla rice milk
1 teaspoon vanilla

3 cups all-purpose flour
1 & 1/2 teaspoons baking powder
1/2 teaspoon salt
6 ounces semi-sweet chocolate
    chips, optional
all-vegetable cooking spray

Cream margarine, peanut butter, and sugars together. Beat in eggs, one at a time. Mix in rice milk and vanilla. Stir in flour, baking power and salt. Stir in 4 ounces chocolate chips. Spread batter into a 13 x 9-inch baking pan coated with cooking spray. Sprinkle remaining chocolate chips evenly over top. Bake in an oven preheated to 350 degrees for 20 to 25 minutes or until golden brown on top. Makes about 2 dozen brownies.

Rocky Road Brownies

1 stick margarine, softened
1 cup sugar
2 eggs
1 teaspoon vanilla extract
1/3 cup cocoa (unsweetened)
1 & 1/2 cups all-purpose flour
1 teaspoon baking soda

1/4 teaspoon salt
1 cup mini-marshmallows
1/2 cup semi-sweet chocolate
    chips
1/2 cup chopped walnuts
all-vegetable cooking spray

Preheat oven to 350 degrees. Cream margarine and sugar together. Beat in eggs. Mix in vanilla, cocoa, flour, baking soda and salt. Pour batter into a 9 x 9-inch baking pan coated with cooking spray. Bake for 25 minutes. Sprinkle marshmallows, chocolate chips and walnuts evenly over top of batter and return to oven for 5 more minutes. Makes 9 brownies.

Lemon Bars

Crust:
1/2 cup sugar
6 tablespoons margarine, softened
1 & 3/4 cups all-purpose flour

Filling:
5 eggs

1 & 1/2 cups sugar
1 tablespoon grated lemon rind
1/2 cup fresh lemon juice
5 tablespoons all-purpose flour
1 teaspoon baking powder
1/4 teaspoon salt
powdered sugar for garnish

Preheat oven to 350 degrees. Mix first three ingredients together until mixture is crumbly (a food processor works well for this). Press mixture into the bottom of a 13 x 9-inch pan and bake for 15 to 18 minutes. Cool.

Beat eggs with an electric mixer until foamy and lemon colored. Add sugar and beat well. Then add lemon rind, lemon juice, flour, baking powder and salt. Beat until well blended. Pour lemon mixture over crust and bake at 350 degrees for 20 to 25 minutes, until set. Cool, then sprinkle powdered sugar. Makes 20-24 bars.

Caramel Orange Bread Pudding

1 tablespoon grated orange rind
1/2 cup orange juice
1/3 cup sugar
4 eggs
2 cups enriched rice milk
1/2 cup brown sugar
2 teaspoons vanilla extract
1/2 teaspoon cinnamon
1/8 teaspoon nutmeg

12 one-inch thick slices of
    French or sourdough bread
    (baguette style)
all-vegetable cooking spray

Topping:
3 tablespoons brown sugar
1/2 teaspoon cinnamon
1 tablespoon margarine

    Combine first three ingredients in a small saucepan. Bring to a boil over medium heat, stirring constantly. Boil until mixture is thickened slightly, about 6-8 minutes. Set aside. Whisk eggs until well blended. Whisk in rice milk, vanilla, cinnamon and nutmeg. Arrange bread slices in a 13 x 9-inch pan coated with cooking spray. Pour cooled orange mixture over the bread, then pour egg mixture over bread. Cover and chill in refrigerator for 1-2 hours, or overnight.

    Preheat oven to 350 degrees. Mix together ingredients for topping until crumbly and sprinkle over top of pudding. Bake for 40 to 45 minutes until golden brown and puffed up. Serve warm, garnish with fresh fruit.

Rice Pudding

5 cups enriched rice milk
1 cup white rice
1/2 cup sugar
2 tablespoons margarine

2 teaspoons ground cinnamon
2 teaspoons vanilla
2 egg yolks
1/2 cup raisins

    Combine 4 cups rice milk, rice, sugar, margarine, and cinnamon in a large saucepan. Cook over medium heat until rice is tender and creamy, stirring frequently. Remove from heat and stir in vanilla and raisins. In a small pan heat remaining 1 cup milk, let simmer while stirring constantly. Whisk in egg yolks and cook an additional 2 minutes. Mix egg mixture into rice mixture. May be served warm or cold.

Cinnamon Raisin Bread Pudding

8 cups cinnamon raisin bread
    cubed
8 eggs, may use egg substitute
1 & 1/2 cups sugar
1/2 cup brown sugar

2 cups enriched rice milk
2 teaspoons vanilla
1/2 teaspoon cinnamon
all-vegetable cooking spray

Preheat oven to 350. Spray a 8 x 11-inch pan with cooking spray. Place bread cubes in pan. Whisk together eggs, rice milk, sugars, vanilla and cinnamon. Pour egg mixture over bread; let sit for 15-20 minutes. Bake for 35 to 40 minutes, until puffed and lightly browned. Serve warm.

Vanilla Cinnamon Pudding

1/4 cup sugar
1 egg
2 cups enriched vanilla rice milk

4 tablespoons tapioca (small size)
1/2 teaspoon ground cinnamon

Whisk above ingredients together in a heavy saucepan over medium-high heat. Continue heating, while stirring constantly, until mixture boils. Remove from heat and cool. Pudding may be served warm or chilled.

Tip: rice milk is thin in texture and does not thicken up easily; thus puddings are more likely to have a heavy saucelike consistency. This pudding is great spooned over fresh fruit, such as strawberries!

Banana Bread Pudding

2 & 1/2 cups enriched vanilla
    rice milk
1/2 cup sugar
1 teaspoon cinnamon
1/2 teaspoon nutmeg

3 eggs, beaten
3 tablespoons brown sugar
2 tablespoons margarine
2 ripe bananas, sliced
4 cups French bread, cubed
all-vegetable cooking spray

Preheat oven to 350 degrees. Whisk milk, eggs, sugar, vanilla, cinnamon, and nutmeg until blended. Add bread and let stand 10-15 minutes.

In a medium skillet, heat margarine and brown sugar. Continue stirring until mixture boils and sugar is dissolved. Add sliced bananas and coat in brown sugar mixture, stirring constantly, 1-2 minutes. Fold bananas into bread mixture and pour into an 8 x 8-inch baking dish coated with cooking spray.

Bake for 45-50 minutes, until pudding is golden brown and set. Serve warm.

Blueberry Cobbler

1 large loaf French or sourdough
    bread, crusts trimmed and
    cubed
    6 eggs
1 cup enriched vanilla rice milk
1/2 cup sugar

1/2 cup brown sugar
2 tablespoons cornstarch
1 teaspoon cinnamon
8 cups blueberries (may be fresh
    or frozen)
all-vegetable cooking spray

Place cubed bread in a large mixing bowl. In a separate large bowl, whisk together eggs and rice milk. Pour over bread mixture to coat, cover, and refrigerate for several hours or overnight.

When ready to bake, mix sugars, cornstarch, and cinnamon in a large mixing bowl. Toss in blueberries to coat. Pour blueberries into a 13 × 9-inch baking dish coated with cooking spray, and top with soaked bread cubes.

Bake in an oven preheated to 425 degrees for 30 to 40 minutes. Serves 8.

Chocolate Chip Zucchini Cake

2 & 1/4 cups all-purpose flour
1/2 cup unsweetened cocoa
1 teaspoon baking soda
1 teaspoon salt
1 stick margarine, softened
1/4 cup canola oil
1 jar #2 baby food prunes
2 eggs (egg substitute may be
    used)

1 teaspoon vanilla
1/2 cup enriched chocolate rice
    milk
2 cups grated zucchini
6 ounces (1 cup) semi-sweet
    chocolate chips
1/2 cup chopped walnuts
all-vegetable cooking spray

Preheat oven to 325 degrees. Spray a 13 x 9-inch pan with cooking spray. Mix flour, cocoa, baking soda and salt together in a medium mixing bowl and set aside. Beat margarine, sugar, oil, and prunes until well blended. Add eggs one at a time, beating well after each addition. Mix in dry ingredients alternately with chocolate rice milk. Beat in vanilla. Stir in grated zucchini until just mixed. Pour batter into prepared pan. Sprinkle chocolate chips and nuts over top. Bake 45-50 minutes until a tester comes out clean. May be served warm or cooled. Great with vanilla frozen rice dessert.

German Chocolate Cake

1/2 cup margarine, softened
4 ounces semi-sweet chocolate
    chips
1 & 1/2 cups sugar
1/2 cup enriched chocolate rice
    milk

2 large eggs
2 & 1/2 cups all-purpose flour
2 teaspoons baking powder
1/4 teaspoon salt
all-vegetable cooking spray

Preheat oven to 350 degrees. Melt margarine and chocolate in a microwave-safe bowl on medium high until melted, about 1 & 1/2 minutes. Stir until all chocolate is melted. Mix in sugar and vanilla, then beat in eggs one at a time. Mix in baking powder and salt, then mix in flour in small amounts alternating with rice milk. Blend well. Pour into a 13 x 9-inch baking pan coated with cooking spray. Bake at 350 degrees for 30 minutes, or until a wooden toothpick inserted in the center comes out clean. Cool cake on a wire rack.

Frosting:

1 cup sugar
1/2 cup brown sugar

2 & 1/2 tablespoons cornstarch
1 & 1/2 cups enriched vanilla
    rice milk
4 tablespoons margarine
1/3 cup flaked sweetened coconut

Mix together sugars and cornstarch in a heavy saucepan. Turn range on to medium heat and whisk in rice milk. Add margarine. Bring to a boil over medium heat and cook for 1 minute, stirring constantly. Remove from heat, add pecans and coconut. May serve warmed over cake slices or spread over entire cake.

Good served with vanilla frozen rice dessert.

Cherry Coffee Cake

1 & 1/2 cups flour
1/2 cup sugar
1/2 teaspoon salt
1/2 teaspoon baking powder
1/4 teaspoon baking soda
1/2 stick margarine

1 egg
3/4 cups enriched rice milk
1 teaspoon vanilla
1 cup fresh, canned, or frozen
    cherries, pitted and chopped
all-vegetable cooking spray

Preheat oven to 350 degrees. Mix dry ingredients together in a large bowl. Add margarine and cut into flour mixture until crumbly. Whisk egg, vanilla and rice milk together in a small bowl and add to flour mixture and stir or mix until smooth. Pour into 13 x 9-inch pan coated with cooking spray. Sprinkle cherries over batter, then top with streusel mixture.

Streusel Mix:

1/4 cup brown sugar
2 tablespoons flour
1/4 teaspoon salt

1/4 teaspoon cinnamon
1/4 teaspoon nutmeg
2 tablespoons margarine
1/4 cup rolled oats
1/2 cup sliced almonds

Mix above ingredients together until well blended and crumbly. Sprinkle evenly over cake batter and cherries. Bake for 45-50 minutes until a toothpick inserted comes out clean, and top is golden brown.

Cinnamon Coffee Cake

1 & 3/4 cups sugar, divided
1/2 cup chopped walnuts
1 tablespoon ground cinnamon
1 tablespoon unsweetened cocoa
3 cups all-purpose flour
1 tablespoon baking powder

1/2 teaspoon salt
1 & 1/2 sticks margarine
4 eggs
2 teaspoons vanilla extract
1 cup enriched rice milk
all-vegetable cooking spray

Preheat oven to 350 degrees. Spray a 10-inch tube pan with cooking spray. Mix 1/2 cups sugar, walnuts, cinnamon and cocoa, and set aside. Mix flour, baking powder, and salt in a large bowl. Beat margarine with an electric mixer until smooth. Beat in remaining sugar. Add eggs, one at a time, beating well after each addition. Add vanilla. Mix in dry ingredients alternately with rice milk until mixture is well blended. Spoon 1/3 of the batter into the pan, then sprinkle 1/2 of the walnut mixture on top. Pour remaining batter in the pan and sprinkle with remaining walnut mixture. With a knife, cut through the batter to swirl in the walnut mixture.

Bake cake for 45-50 minutes, until tester comes out clean. Cool. Loosen cake with knife around the edges of the pan before unmolding. About 12 servings.

Peach Upside-Down Cake

2 peaches, skinned and sliced
    (about 16 slices)
1 tablespoon margarine, melted
1/2 cup packed brown sugar
2 tablespoons chopped walnuts
1 1/4 cups all-purpose flour
1/3 cup rolled oats
1 teaspoon cinnamon
1/2 teaspoon ginger

2/3 cup granulated sugar
3/4 teaspoon baking powder
1/2 teaspoon baking soda
1/4 teaspoon salt
4 tablespoons margarine, soft-
    ened
1 large egg
1 teaspoon vanilla
1/2 cup enriched rice milk

Preheat oven to 350 degrees. Coat the bottom of a 9-inch round cake pan with melted margarine. Sprinkle brown sugar and walnuts over top of margarine. Arrange peach slices over top of brown sugar and walnut mixture. Set aside. Combine flour, oats, cinnamon, ginger, sugar, baking powder, soda and salt in a medium bowl. Add margarine and cream into mixture. Beat in egg, then stir in vanilla and rice milk until batter is smooth. Pour into prepared pan and bake for 30 to 35 minutes or until a toothpick comes out clean. Allow cake to cool in pan for 5 to 10 minutes, then loosen edges and invert onto a serving plate. Serve warm.